Gay Men Living with Chronic Illnesses and Disabilities: From Crisis to Crossroads

Gay Men Living with Chronic Illnesses and Disabilities: From Crisis to Crossroads has been co-published simultaneously as *Journal of Gay & Lesbian Social Services,* Volume 17, Number 2 2004.

Gay Men Living with Chronic Illnesses and Disabilities: From Crisis to Crossroads

Benjamin Lipton, MSW
Editor

Gay Men Living with Chronic Illnesses and Disabilities: From Crisis to Crossroads has been co-published simultaneously as *Journal of Gay & Lesbian Social Services,* Volume 17, Number 2 2004.

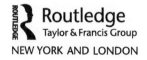

Routledge
Taylor & Francis Group

NEW YORK AND LONDON

First published by
The Haworth Press, Inc.
10 Alice Street
Binghamton, N Y 13904-1580

This edition published 2011 by Routledge

Routledge
Taylor & Francis Group
711 Third Avenue
New York, NY 10017

Routledge
Taylor & Francis Group
2 Park Square, Milton Park
Abingdon, Oxon OX14 4RN

Gay Men Living with Chronic Illnesses and Disabilities: From Crisis to Crossroads has been co-published simultaneously as *Journal of Gay & Lesbian Social Services*, Volume 17, Number 2 2004.

Cover design by Lora Wiggins

Library of Congress Cataloging-in-Publication Data

Gay men living with chronic illnesses and disabilities : from crisis to crossroads / Benjamin Lipton, editor.
    p. cm.
    Published also as v. 17, no. 2, 2004, of the Journal of gay & lesbian social services.
    Includes bibliographical references and index.
    ISBN 1-56023-335-4 (hard cover : alk. paper) – ISBN 1-56023-336-2 (soft cover : alk. paper)
    1. Gay men–Services for. 2. Chronically ill–Services for. 3. Gay men–Health and hygiene. 4. Gay men–Medical care. 5. Older gay men–Medical care. I. Lipton, Benjamin. II. Journal of gay & lesbian social services.
HV1449.G39 2004
362.196'044'008664–dc22
                                                 2004017973

To Steven . . . who, when it comes right down to it, defines wonderful.

And to gay men everywhere who live each day with chronic illnesses and disabilities.

Gay Men Living with Chronic Illnesses and Disabilities: From Crisis to Crossroads

CONTENTS

About the Contributors   xvii

Preface   xix
Eric Rofes

Gay Men Living with Non-HIV Chronic Illnesses   1
Benjamin Lipton

Gay Men Living with Chronic Illness or Disability:
A Sociocultural, Minority Group Perspective on Mental Health   25
William F. Hanjorgiris
Joseph F. Rath
John H. O'Neill

The Gay Male Gaze: Body Image Disturbance
and Gender Oppression Among Gay Men   43
Mitchell J. Wood

The Multidimensional Challenge of Psychotherapy
with HIV Positive Gay Men   63
Ronald J. Frederick

Resistance and Resilience: The Untold Story
of Gay Men Aging with Chronic Illnesses   81
John Genke

The Impact of a Non-HIV Chronic Illness on Professional
Practice: Personal and Professional
Considerations of a Psychotherapist   97
Charles P. Isola

Index   111

ABOUT THE EDITOR

Benjamin Lipton, MSW, is a clinical social worker and supervisor in private practice in New York City. In addition, he is a consultant to GLBT-identified and mainstream social service and health care organizations on issues related to mental health, chronic illness, patient support and sexuality. Mr. Lipton is the former Director of Clinical Services at Gay Men's Health Crisis (GMHC). He is an adjunct faculty member in Social Work at New York University where he is also completing his doctoral studies. His work on clinical practice with gay men and people living with chronic illnesses has been presented at numerous conferences and symposia and has been published in edited volumes, academic journals, and popular periodicals. He received a Master of Social Work degree from New York University and a BA from Yale University. Mr. Lipton serves on the editorial board of the *Journal of Gay & Lesbian Social Services*.

About the Contributors

Ronald J. Frederick, PhD, LP, has been Supervising Psychologist for Park House Adult Day Health/Day Treatment Program of Abbott Northwestern Hospital in Minneapolis, MN, since 1998. He holds a doctoral degree in clinical psychology from Fairleigh Dickinson University and completed a postdoctoral fellowship in Medical Psychology and AIDS at the AIDS Center Program of St. Luke's-Roosevelt Hospital Center in New York City. In addition to maintaining a private practice in Minneapolis, Dr. Frederick has presented numerous papers, seminars and workshops, has written articles and book chapters on an array of mental health issues, and is actively involved in training clinicians from a variety of different disciplines.

John Genke, MSW, CSW, is Senior Social Worker at Senior Action in a Gay Environment (SAGE) in New York City. SAGE offers a full range of social services, advocacy, and socialization opportunities to senior members of the lesbian, gay, bisexual and transgender community in the New York metropolitan area. He is a member of NASW and The Association for the Advancement for Social Work with Groups.

William F. Hanjorgiris received a PhD in counseling psychology from Fordham University. He currently maintains a private psychotherapy practice in NYC and is on staff at Rivington House–The Nicholas A. Rango Healthcare Facility. His research and clinical interests focus on gay male identity development (coming out), masculinity, chronic illness, and trauma. He is a contributing author to the *Handbook of Counseling and Psychotherapy with Lesbian, Gay, and Bisexual Clients*.

Charles P. Isola began a master's program in social work when he was forty years old. Previously, he worked in the securities industry. In addition to his MSW, he holds an MA in French and an MA in education as well as a group training certificate from the E.G.P.S. He is currently retired.

John H. O'Neill received a PhD in rehabilitation counselor education from Syracuse University and is a Nationally Certified Rehabilitation Counselor. Currently, he is Professor and Coordinator of Counselor Education at Hunter College, City University of New York. His research focuses on the community integration and employment of two distinct populations: individuals living with HIV/AIDS and people who have experienced a traumatic brain injury.

Joseph F. Rath is a licensed psychologist and a research scientist at New York University School of Medicine's Rusk Institute of Rehabilitation Medicine. He earned his PhD in counseling psychology from Fordham University. He has done research and clinical work with people with disabilities since 1993, when he was the recipient of a National Institutes of Health Fellowship in Rehabilitation Research. An adjunct faculty member and clinical supervisor in the Department of Counseling and Clinical Psychology at Columbia University Teachers College, he maintains a private psychotherapy practice in New York City.

Eric Rofes is Assistant Professor of Education at Humboldt State University in Arcata, California, where he teaches courses on community organizing, gay issues in schools, and social foundations of education. He earned his doctorate in social and cultural studies from UC Berkeley Graduate School of Education. He is the author of 10 books, including *Dry Bones Breathe: Gay Men Creating Post-AIDS Identities and Cultures* (The Haworth Press, Inc., 1998). He currently engages in grassroots organizing on gay men's health in the United States. Dr. Rofes is the founder of the Boston Lesbian & Gay Political Alliance and the executive director of the Los Angeles Gay and Lesbian Community Services Center and the Shanti Project, San Francisco's pioneering AIDS service group.

Mitchell J. Wood is a psychotherapist in private practice in New York City. He is affiliated with the Columbia University Center for Gay and Lesbian Mental Health and has been an adjunct faculty member at the Hunter College School of Social Work. He received his Master in Divinity from Union Theological Seminary and his Master in Social Work from Columbia University. As the Director of Mental Health Programs at Goodwill Industries, Mr. Wood developed and administered psychosocial and vocational rehabilitation programs for homeless adults with psychiatric disabilities. He is currently in the dissertation phase of the doctoral program at the School of Social Work at New York University.

Preface

Eric Rofes

I have spent much of the past five years organizing national summits focused on the health and wellness of gay male communities. Working with a team of collaborators from throughout the United States, we've organized three national summits drawing together activists, health providers, researchers, and HIV prevention leaders for discussion and debate about promising new directions intended to support and strengthen our communities and subcultures. Over 20 local and regional summits have taken place, not only in cities such as New York and San Francisco, but also in rural Georgia; Missoula, Montana; Salt Lake City, Utah; and Raleigh North Carolina. New gay men's health projects have recently opened in Seattle, Philadelphia, Tucson, and San Francisco, and organizers throughout the West are considering adopting multi-issue, multicultural efforts in order to strengthen their work with gay men. All of a sudden, something called the "gay men's health movement" is on the lips of policy makers, AIDS activists, and journalists alike.

This is a moment of great rethinking. Our efforts are part of a broader movement intended to shift the focus of gay community discourse and institutional work away from HIV-centric approaches and into holistic and multi-issue health work. We are not ostriches, sticking our heads in the sand to avoid continuing work on HIV. We are aware that HIV continues to infect gay and bisexual men of all colors and generations and that, as a community, we face strong challenges in this area. Yet we've realized that the old approaches developed during the crisis moment of AIDS in the United States no longer work as effectively as they once

[Haworth co-indexing entry note]: "Preface." Rofes, Eric. Co-published simultaneously in *Journal of Gay & Lesbian Social Services* (Harrington Park Press, an imprint of The Haworth Press, Inc.) Vol. 17, No. 2, 2004, pp. xxiii-xxvi; and: *Gay Men Living with Chronic Illnesses and Disabilities: From Crisis to Crossroads* (ed: Benjamin Lipton) Harrington Park Press, an imprint of The Haworth Press, Inc., 2004, pp. xix- xxii. Single or multiple copies of this article are available for a fee from The Haworth Document Delivery Service [1-800-HAWORTH, 9:00 a.m. - 5:00 p.m. (EST). E-mail address: docdelivery@haworthpress.com].

xix

did. We've realized that we need to re-envision what it means to work on gay men's health issues. This involves both reconceptualizing our work in a broader fashion, and re-politicizing our work, as we face the ignorance, hostility, and disdain of a new, rising homophobia in our nation.

This groundbreaking volume suggests useful paths forward as we struggle to reimagine what community health and wellness might look like for gay men. Focusing on the psychosocial experiences of gay men living with chronic illnesses *other than* HIV, Lipton's article provides a theoretical and practical framework for understanding the pervasive impact of HIV on our conceptions of both health and illness. He challenges us to resist the social construction that we live in a bifurcated world where gay men are either HIV negative and healthy, or HIV positive and sick. He argues instead for the development of more nuanced understandings of health and illness among gay men, not only related to HIV, but also the myriad of other health concerns and disabilities that our communities face.

What does it mean, for example, that throughout the nation, gay men are living with all kinds of chronic diseases and disabling conditions, yet the only solid community health infrastructure we've developed is focused on HIV/AIDS? As more and more gay men move through midlife into old age, how have we failed to produce a support system, parallel to the current HIV system of care, that is focused on aging, chronic illness and disability? Why have we created institutions, identities, and subcultures solely around HIV, rather than, for example, hepatitis, diabetes, heart disease and cancer? The powerful essays that follow both directly and indirectly explore these questions and make it clear that HIV is only one challenge among many facing the men in our communities.

As we raise questions about current cultural definitions of HIV in the United States, we face huge resistance from many health advocates and gay activists who challenge our belief that it may be helpful for all gay men, whether they are living with HIV or not, to reconceptualize HIV as a chronic illness. Some who oppose this move are clinging to a specific epidemic moment that provided gay men with an odd sort of heroism in the mind of America; our first decade of AIDS work brought with it great visibility that we successfully marshaled to show ourselves to be a community that faced the challenge of AIDS head-on. Others are locked in an understanding of HIV disease that makes it unique and different from all other forms of chronic illness; they refuse to see parallels and continue to fight to preserve services that have been granted to people with HIV, but not to those with other forms of disabling illness. Frederick's article bravely addresses the current, conflicted moment in the sociocultural evolution of HIV from the perspective of a psychologist working with gay men living with HIV at a Midwestern adult day health center.

This volume explores key issues about gay men and disability that have not, unfortunately, been widely addressed in our communities. There was a moment during the first decade of AIDS when gay men's communities seemed on the brink of having a broad conversation about disability and ableism, and about the ways in which gay male cultures presented barriers to men with disabilities. It became common to see men with a range of disabling conditions at gay events, neighborhoods, and commercial establishments. Taking a lesson from a much deeper conversation occurring among lesbian feminists, gay men began welcoming sign language interpreters to our events, creating social programs and low-cost cultural events for disabled men, and finding creative ways to ensure access to community institutions to the increasing number of gay men in wheelchairs or walking with canes. We began to understand the need to recognize able-bodied status as one of privilege, and often temporary privilege at that.

This moment seemed to end abruptly, however, as new treatments allowed more men with HIV to function more fully in their everyday lives, and the number of men who were recognizably disabled diminished in gay communities. As younger men moved into prominent positions in community life–men whose knowledge of the height of the epidemic could only be secondhand, through films like *Philadelphia*, oral histories, or books about the early days of AIDS–a politicized awareness of disability issues seemed to disappear from the pages of gay newspapers and discussions at gay conferences. More recently, activism by queer and/or disabled people has revived this discussion. In this volume, Hanjorgiris and his colleagues employ a social constructivist perspective to add important theoretical and practical dialogue to the reemerging conversation about gay men and disability. Hopefully, it will not take years for mainstream health advocates and service providers to understand its relevance to nurturing community life.

Credit goes to Benjamin Lipton and his collaborators for opening up vital questions now facing gay men's communities. In fact, this volume cuts to the heart of the question of community for gay men of my generation and the one before. Many of us distanced ourselves from our families of origin and our hometowns as we embraced identities that were–at that time–confusing and problematic to much of America. Instead, we forged new linkages, created new forms of kinship, and developed meaningful rituals that sustained us through the joys and struggles of life. What responsibilities does "community" have to gay men who have aged out of youth-oriented gay culture? When we face chronic illness, what can community offer us? Or are we expected to rely on heterosexist medical and social services, and return home to those same families of origin for care? Genke, a social worker at Senior Action in a Gay Environment (SAGE), explores the psychosocial challenges that older gay men must contend with as they deal with illness and disability in our ageist culture. Cutting just as close to the bone, Wood's article on body image disturbance among gay men explores the pervasive impact that our oppressive, gendered construction of the body has on the availability of our communities to make space for and value difference and diversity, whether related to age, illness, disability or any other social phenomenon. Finally, Isola, a social worker who was diagnosed with a chronic illness unrelated to HIV while working in an HIV/AIDS unit of a major hospital, reminds us through his personal narrative of the very real lives that are affected by the ways in which we do and do *not* build representative and supportive communities for gay men living with debilitating health concerns.

The bottom line is this: We need to shift to a more complex and comprehensive understanding of health and illness, especially in the ways these concepts affect gay men. Those of us who are building theory, conducting research, and providing services to gay men need to challenge the HIV-infected vs. healthy binary that still informs much of our thinking. The alternative is to valorize a divisive project of categorization that marginalizes HIV positive men as uniquely and deathly ill, while rendering invisible the many men with non-HIV-related health concerns who live amongst us and deserve to share equally in community life.

This important volume opens up this conversation in a useful and progressive manner. It's time for the rest of us to join in.

Gay Men Living
with Non-HIV Chronic Illnesses

Benjamin Lipton

SUMMARY. For reasons embedded in historical, social, cultural and biological phenomena, the sociocultural experiences of gay men living with chronic illnesses *other* than HIV have remained unexamined within gay communities, within gay affirmative medical and social services, and within broader, heterosexually focused medical and social service systems. As a result, the specific needs of these men are largely undefined and potentially unmet. This article focuses a lens of inquiry on the psychosocial issues and social service needs of gay men living with chronic illnesses other than HIV, offers recommendations for providing services that respond proactively to the specific needs of these men, and advocates for more inclusive and comprehensive social service and health care systems. *[Article copies available for a fee from The Haworth Document Delivery Service: 1-800-HAWORTH. E-mail address: <docdelivery@ haworthpress.com> Website: <http://www.HaworthPress.com> © 2004 by The Haworth Press, Inc. All rights reserved.]*

KEYWORDS. Chronic illness, gay men, HIV negative, health care, social services, stigma

---

Benjamin Lipton, MSW, is affiliated with the New York University Ehrenkranz School of Social Work. Address correspondence to: 156 Fifth Avenue, Suite 1116, New York, NY 10010 (E-mail: benjaminlipton@aol.com).

[Haworth co-indexing entry note]: "Gay Men Living with Non-HIV Chronic Illnesses." Lipton, Benjamin. Co-published simultaneously in *Journal of Gay & Lesbian Social Services* (Harrington Park Press, an imprint of The Haworth Press, Inc.) Vol. 17, No. 2, 2004, pp. 1-23; and: *Gay Men Living with Chronic Illnesses and Disabilities: From Crisis to Crossroads* (ed: Benjamin Lipton) Harrington Park Press, an imprint of The Haworth Press, Inc., 2004, pp. 1-23. Single or multiple copies of this article are available for a fee from The Haworth Document Delivery Service [1-800-HAWORTH, 9:00 a.m. - 5:00 p.m. (EST). E-mail address: docdelivery@haworthpress.com].

http://www.haworthpress.com/web/JGLSS
© 2004 by The Haworth Press, Inc. All rights reserved.
Digital Object Identifier: 10.1300/J041v17n02_01

For the past two decades, the gay community has been immersed in an encompassing transformation to address the impact of the HIV virus. As a result, HIV has become the hub from which responses to the medical and psychosocial concerns of gay men now radiate. While exemplary systems of psychosocial support and biomedical breakthroughs of the past decade are tributes to a collaborative single-mindedness and dedication to fighting HIV, this fight has also left in its wake communal trauma of immense proportions (Rofes, 1996). Some sequelae to the trauma of the HIV epidemic are readily apparent; others ripple much more subtly beneath the surface. One significant yet heretofore undocumented result of the HIV epidemic may be the near invisibility of gay men living with *non*-HIV chronic illnesses (NHIVCIs). Because the social response to AIDS has been entirely consuming, it has left little psychological room and even fewer financial or scientific resources with which to evaluate and explore the biopsychosocial impact of sexual orientation on gay men living with *other* health concerns. This invisibility is apparent both within the domains of gay culture and gay affirmative medical and social services, as well as within the broader, heterosexually focused medical and social service communities targeting people living with a broad range of chronic health concerns.

INCIDENCE AND PREVALENCE
OF CHRONIC ILLNESSES AMONG GAY MEN

Based on various sources of epidemiological statistics, many researchers conclude that more than half of all American adults have a chronic health condition (Landis, 1991; Shuman, 1996). LaPlante and Carlson (1996) argue that between 8.5 percent and 17 percent of the U.S. population is disabled due to illness. No demographic data has ever been collected on the proportion of these men and woman who are gay or lesbian. However, according to current data, the number of *publicly self-identified* gay men and lesbians is between 2.8% and 9.1% of the overall adult population in the United States (Laumann et al., 1994). Importantly, the authors note that these numbers are likely to be under-representative due to the limited ability of survey research to capture sensitive information from sexual minorities. If we apply these percentages to data on the overall number of adult Americans living with chronic health conditions, it can be inferred that somewhere between 366,950 and 9,353,700 gay men and lesbians are currently living with a chronic health issues (U.S. Census Bureau, 2002). Moreover, even if we subtract from this number the HIV positive U.S. men who have sex with men, then it is likely that there are *at least* hundreds of thousands, and possibly several millions, of gay men living with chronic illnesses *other* than HIV in the United States (Center for Disease Control, 2002).

A BIOPSYCHOSOCIAL DEFINITION OF NON-HIV CHRONIC ILLNESS (NHIVCIs) FOR GAY MEN

Diseases are bio-physiological phenomena that are described in terms of scientific observation and inference. Illnesses, on the other hand, are described not only in terms of science, but also in terms of psychology and social interaction. They represent the entirety of the lived experiences of disease processes (Shuman, 1996; Sontag, 1978, 1988). Chronic physical illnesses, in particular, represent the biopsychosocial experience of living with disease processes that are perpetual, permanently affecting and disruptive to the expected human life cycle (Garrett & Weisman, 2001). Diagnosis of a chronic illness is often difficult, and once identified, the disease course is frequently hard to predict. It may be slow and insidious, fast and immediately catastrophic, or cycle through recurring episodes of exacerbation and remission. Exacerbation of disease processes may cause irrevocable, pathological changes that require ongoing observation, medical intervention and rehabilitation efforts. Syndromes may include the loss of physical and/or mental capacity and create dramatic changes in the level of functioning. People living with chronic illnesses experience incurable, frequently debilitating physical impairment with the potential for either temporary or permanent physical disabilities, disfigurement, and shortened life span (Goodheart & Lansing, 1996). While this broad definition is well represented in the literature (Cujpers, 1998; Joachim & Acorn, 2000; Lewis, 1999), the impetus to create a generic definition of chronic illness in order to construct a broadly applicable understanding of the phenomenon may easily obscure the very reason that these illnesses are so challenging for those who live with them. Namely, that they are insistently *particular* regarding prognosis, extent of functional incapacitation, visibility, and amenability to treatment (Donoghue & Siegel, 2001).

Uncertainty and unpredictability are unifying themes for people living with chronic illnesses (Shuman, 1996). Adjustment to a diagnosis and subsequent illness management depend upon previous levels of psychological functioning, beliefs about the meaning of illness, and available social and environmental supports, e.g., access to care, financial assistance, and social support networks (Goin, 1990). As with the normative response to any crisis, psychological regression frequently accompanies both diagnosis and subsequent episodes of disease exacerbation. Fear of loss of control, dependency, separation and loss, shame and guilt, anger, isolation, and sexual anxiety are frequently provoked by the experience of a disease run rampant in a body out of control. These developmental conflicts may cause disillusionment and disruption in baseline functioning (Garrett & Weisman, 2001).

From the very early moments of emerging awareness that "something is wrong" with one's body, the diagnostic process related to chronic illnesses, combined with the potential for minimizing of subjective internal symptoms by medical providers, can lead people to feel responsible for their symptoms on the one hand, or a false sense of control over their illness on the other (Donoghue & Siegel, 2001).

For gay men, in particular, the cultural and psychological specter of HIV hovers over and further compounds the diagnostic process of any physiological problem. Nearly every gay man, whether through personal experience or vicarious cultural transmission, has been steeped in the sequelae to the destruction and dying related to HIV (Rofes, 1996). As a result, if HIV is ruled out as a medical concern, survivor guilt may obscure the core emotional reaction of a gay man to learning that he has a different chronic illness. This may be manifest in a number of ways. A man may feel unentitled to claim a "sick" label if his disease is less deadly than HIV. He may feel ashamed of his inability to tolerate his symptoms. He may feel deserving of this illness as compensation for not contracting HIV. Or he may be fused defensively to a rationalization that "at least it's not AIDS" (Lipton, 1997, 1998). If, on the other hand, a man is already diagnosed with HIV and then receives an additional diagnosis of another illness–which is now occurring with increasing frequency secondary to anti-retroviral combination therapy–then this new diagnosis may be psychologically overwhelming and exceed one's capacity to cope. Often, a secondary diagnosis to HIV can feed, or revive, a depressive cognitive feedback loop of inevitable demise, leading to the exacerbation of feelings of anxiety related to physical vulnerability and an abandonment of hope (Paradis, 1993).

The HIV epidemic has ruptured the understanding of a continuum of wellness within the gay community. It has led gay men and those who provide them with medical and social services to paint a picture of health and illness in broad strokes of life or death. For gay men and many of their service providers, HIV now seems to be the unconsciously accepted litmus test of health. Either you have HIV and are "sick,"or you are HIV negative and therefore "healthy." The prevalence of this perspective both reflects and reinforces the felt experience of gay men living with a myriad of other health concerns: they are absent from the professional and social discourses of the gay community (Lipton, 1998).

It is important to note here that with few exceptions, gay men have to navigate this psychological tightrope of diagnosis and management of their diseases in professional relationships with medical providers who are frequently heterosexual and/or hetero-normative (Dean, 2000). Sensitivity on the part of these providers to the particular cultural history regarding how gay men make sense of illness as well as the expectation of stigmatization that gay men bring to the examination room, especially in geographic areas with smaller openly gay populations, is rare. Moreover, this need for attunement must encompass not only the legacy of homophobia and heterosexism within medical services–something which providers are becoming increasingly aware of (Gay & Lesbian Medical Association, 1999)–but also must reflect an understanding of the immense impact that HIV has had on how men make sense of *all other* health concerns.

Exploring the internalization of HIV for gay men living with chronic illnesses suggests a fundamental difference between their experiences and those of heterosexuals living with the same illnesses. While, with few exceptions, illness is *entirely* denied in heterosexual culture, the daily reality of illness *has been* a part of the fabric of life for contemporary gay men for the past two decades–but *only* through the lens of HIV (Sontag, 1988; Rofes, 1996). The significance of this phenomenon for gay men living with chronic illnesses–and particularly if they are HIV-negative–seems powerful. As a result of the gay community's response to HIV, many gay men are aware of the possibility of and need for sick people to receive meaningful and *culturally competent* concrete and emotional support. They see it in the impressive, comprehensive systems of care set up for gay men and other minority groups living with HIV. They see it each time they open a gay (and sometimes mainstream) periodical and read an advertisement for a gay event where part of the proceeds will go to an HIV-related charity. At the same time, doors to these HIV-related services are usually closed to gay men living with illness other than HIV, and equivalent services are not provided elsewhere.

As a result, a gay man living with NHIVCIs must rely on organizations that address the general, heterosexual population living with his specific disease (e.g., the American Cancer Society, the Muscular Sclerosis Society, etc.). Not surprisingly, these organizations are frequently heterosexist, either by benign neglect or by clear intention (often due to biased funding sources), and fail to respond to the specific needs of gay people (Dean et al., 2000).

Gay men living with NHIVCIs appear to live in a no-man's land as they are forced to straddle two communities: their gay peers on the one hand, and their (frequently) heterosexual medical providers and heterosexist patient support organizations on the other. They are not reflected in the gay cultural norms and iconography that shot up defensively in the wake of HIV and fetishize physical development and invulnerability (Rofes, 1996; Sadownick, 1996; Signorile, 1997). Neither are they reflected in the heterosexual cultural narratives and iconography of mainstream medical and psychosocial services (Joachim & Acorn, 2000). Instead, gay men living with NHIVCIs are displaced to the margins in terms of psychological concerns, physical health and appearance, and sexual attractiveness by both the heterosexual majority and by their own sexual minority group.

THE SOCIAL CONSTRUCTION
OF ILLNESS AND GAY IDENTITY

To date, the only body of theoretical literature related to social services that describes the interplay of male sexual orientation with the experience of living with a chronic physical illness is the literature on HIV/AIDS (see Martin & Hunter, 2001, for an extensive annotated bibliography on this subject). This literature also documents the embeddedness of HIV within a unique political and sociocultural matrix and argues that living with HIV cannot be generalized meaningfully to what it means to be living with other illnesses in contemporary society (Cadwell, 1990; Sontag, 1988). In the absence of any theory that directly addresses the impact on gay men of chronic illnesses other than HIV, how can we theorize about the psychosocial experiences of gay men living with those other illnesses? A useful jumping-off point may be to develop our understanding of the ways in which our culture has made and ascribed meaning separately and synergistically to the concepts of chronic illness and homosexuality. The interplay of these two concepts over the last several decades has profoundly impacted society in general and cuts to the heart of the social and psychological factors with which gay men who are chronically ill must currently contend.

The concepts of chronic illness and gay identity are slippery social constructions, informed perhaps by biological manifestations but dependent for their current meanings upon contemporary social conceptualizations regarding sickness and sexuality (Chauncey, 1994; Herek, 1990; Sontag, 1978, 1988). The development of their definitions takes place within a complex series of social interactions between scientists, physicians, patients, insurance companies, government agencies, religious organizations, media manufacturers, and others.

Herek (1990) suggests that the social construction of illness typically includes four components. First, the *origin* of an illness is identified. Then, *responsibility* for the disease is assigned simultaneously with the construction and assignment of the *role* of the person living with the disease (e.g., innocent victim or moral degenerate, dangerous or benign; hero or predator). Finally, responsibility for a *cure* is assigned. During this process, the culture at large imbues a disease with meaning by integrating it into a larger ontology. Some may construct a vision of compassion or disdain based upon moral conviction. Others may construct a plan of social action or inaction based upon pragmatism and the rational evaluation of the impact of illness on an individual and/or society. Ultimately, the way one understands and responds to illness is the result of the complex interplay of personal epistemology and hegemonic societal constructs of meaning (Herek, 1990).

Perhaps no clearer contemporary example of the embeddedness of illness within a sociocultural context can be found than in the journey that the construct of homosexuality continues to take across our cultural landscape. Until 1973, homosexuality was classified as a mental disorder requiring psychiatric intervention (Abelove, 1993). Applying Herek's (1990) model of illness construction to homosexuality prior to its declassification, we can see that the *origin* of homosexuality was assigned to derailment in early childhood development; that *responsibility* for homosexuality was assigned to the families (and particularly the mothers) of homosexual individuals; that the *role* of the "sick" homosexual was defined as stunted, degenerate, and dangerous; and that *responsibility for cure* lay entirely in the lap of the identified ill person (Frommer, 1995). Reflective of the sociocultural milieu, social institutions did their part to reinforce and sustain this moralistic, quasi-religious construction of homosexuality (Abelove, 1993).

With the advent of sweeping social reforms in the 1960s, however, cultural definitions of normalcy and acceptability began to shift. Fueled by the civil rights victories of other oppressed minorities, advocates for a scientific conceptualization of sexual orientation advocated for the recognition among the medical establishment that homosexuality was a normative and healthy line of sexual development (Bayer, 1981; Krajeski,

1986). They fought to disentangle the previous attachment of moral judgment from the concept of sexual orientation. New affirmative constructions of the identities of *gay* and *lesbian* entered the sociocultural discourse to challenge established, pathology-based beliefs (Chauncey, 1994). Importantly, these new identity constructs were not simply more benign contemporary substitutes for earlier negative definitions of what it is to be a homosexual. In other words, the homosexual man of old has not simply been replaced by the gay man of today. Rather, social changes have dramatically expanded the ways in which we understand sexual orientation to include much more than sexual behavior. For example, earlier constructions of homosexuality did not include discourses about such issues as meaningful dyadic relationships, marriage possibilities, child rearing, insurance benefits, and political affiliations, etc. As a result of this historical shift still in process, two conflicting constructions of homosexuality, one rooted in a disease model and the other based upon a demand for understanding homosexuality as normative, play off each other and contribute to the current ambivalent sociocultural moment with regard to making sense of sexual orientation.

As the debate over the validity of homosexual orientation was generating new cultural conceptions with regard to sexuality during 1970s and early 1980s, another closely linked transformation of meaning was also taking place in the arena of disease (Sontag, 1988). The advent of the AIDS epidemic reawakened dormant societal fears about illness. As gay men began to die in painful and ugly ways by a disease transmitted through sex, cultural beliefs about homosexuality as a degenerate practice or "lifestyle" linked up with cultural anxieties about disease and led to a resurgence of socially sanctioned stigmatizing of those living with HIV (Herek, 1990; Sontag, 1988). The stigma attached to AIDS as an illness was layered upon preexisting stigma regarding both illness and sexual orientation and, to a great extent, equated with it (Herek, 1990). Thus, the advent of the AIDS epidemic has served not only to rekindle phobic responses to those who are ill, but also to those who are gay. The century old connection between homosexuality and degeneracy, built upon long-standing, religiously based views of morality, breathed new life into efforts by some to pathologize homosexuality.

STIGMA AND GAY MEN LIVING WITH NHIVCIs

What, then, are the implications of these ambivalent, shifting social constructions of homosexuality and illness on the psychological experiences of contemporary gay men who are facing the challenge of living with chronic illnesses other than HIV? One useful answer to this question lies in an exploration of theory related to stigma and minority stress. The current cultural conflict over how to understand both homosexuality and illness is not only alive in the broader, sociocultural discourse, but also informs the individual psychological experiences of gay men residing within that discourse. In gay men, the pull toward the construction of homosexuality as deviant and immoral lives side by side with the push toward an assertive, affirming identity (Cornett, 1993). In other words, the legacy of heterosexism and homophobia leave gay men vulnerable to the threat of stigma, whether ill or relatively healthy. Moreover, for a gay man who is ill, the stigma surrounding a homosexual orientation is compounded not only by the cultural stigma ascribed to all diseases, but also by the unique shadow of AIDS-related stigma that the legacy of HIV casts on a *gay* man who is living with *any* illness nowadays. Thus, a gay man living with a NHIVCI must negotiate a complex and at times chaotic web of stigmatized identities. Multiple, concomitant exposures to stigmatizing social interactions, both as a gay man *and* as someone who is sick with a "heterosexualized" (e.g., not HIV-related) illness, leaves him with challenging psychosocial tasks with regard to maintaining a positive self-identity and locating an affirmative social environment.

In what is perhaps the best known and most enduring theoretical discussion of the concept of stigma, Goffman (1963) defined it as "an attribute that is deeply discrediting within a particular social interaction" (p. 3). The stigma ascribed to people of minority sexual orientations is well documented in every body of literature. Words such as homophobia, internalized homophobia, and heterosexism generously pepper writings on the psychological and social theory of homosexuality in an effort to conceptualize and describe the interpersonal dynamic of hatred toward gay people and its resulting impact on both homosexual and heterosexual segments of the population (Sears & Williams, 1997). The process of coming out, now widely accepted as a normal task of development for gay men and lesbians and often framed as a celebration of self-affirmation, nonetheless implicitly speaks to the legacy of shame and self-hatred that a gay person must work through if they are to achieve some level of self-acceptance. Without gay stigma, coming out would not be necessary.

The process of stigmatization is also very much alive for people living with chronic illnesses (Sontag, 1978; Joachim & Acorn, 2000). Phillips (1990) conceives of labeling as an inevitable, negative outcome of disability. People with illnesses and disabilities in our culture are considered "damaged goods" or to have a "spoiled identity" (Goffman, 1963). This stigma is caused not by the disability itself, but by the difference between what is socially desirable and what in fact *is* for a person who appears outside the norm (Cadwell, 1992; Herek, 1990; Joachim & Acorn; 2000; Meyer, 1995). Theorizing a parallel to heterosexism, Thorne (1993) argues that a person with a visible disability or chronic illness is actually rendered *invisible* by the reactions of others. Others conceptualize a process of stigmatization by which people react to health disparities with both overt and covert discrimination (Herek, 1990). This process includes the construction of a belief system that enables people to invoke labels such as "cripple" or "defective" by rationalizing that those being labeled pose a danger to the majority. Their physical differences, labeled as shortcomings and linked to moral failing, work to dehumanize a sick person and mitigate the potential for guilt feelings of those who stigmatize (Sontag, 1988). Others maintain that the sight of or knowledge that someone is chronically ill induces vulnerability and fear of being afflicted with the same illness (Sontag, 1988). Thus, through the social phenomena of stigma, the ill–like gay men–become scapegoats who must hold the hostile projections of cultural anxieties regarding health, morality and mortality.

It is important to recognize here that the specific impact of stigma on gay men living with NHIVCIs cannot be explained accurately simply by combining the application of stigma theory related to homosexuality with its application to chronic illness. Doing so fails to capture the synergistic effects of living with these two identities simultaneously at this particular cultural moment in the history of our society at large, and our gay communities in particular. First, these men are gay within a heterosexually biased, frequently homophobic society. Then, they are chronically ill within an illness-phobic society and are seeking help within a heterosexually focused health care establishment. At the same time, they are gay men living with "the wrong" illnesses within their sexual minority group that is, in fact, accepting of a different illness, namely HIV. While gay men are familiar with and have made psychological space for the recognition of and destigmatization of HIV, no space seems to be left over to acknowledge and destigmatize the broad range of other chronic health concerns facing gay men today. If anything, a counter-phobic response to the mortal fear and massive devastation brought about by the HIV epidemic seems to have further cemented the denial of physical vulnerability among so many gay men (Rofes, 1996; Sadownick, 1996). So while HIV has in many ways become an accept-

able illness for gay men, other illnesses remain both consciously disavowed and unconsciously denied.

MINORITY STATUS AND MINORITY STRESS

The cumulative impact of living as a gay man with a NHIVCI is to
live under the constant burden of psychosocial stress derived from the
stigma of a compounded minority status. Brooks (1981) aptly defines
this phenomenon as minority stress. The concept of minority stress is
based on the premise that majority groups subject members of minority
groups such as gay people and those who are chronically ill to chronic
stress related to coping with stigmatized identities. This conceptualization is not based upon one congruous psychological or social theory, but
is inferred from several theoretical constructs, all of which posit that the
juxtaposition of minority and dominant values results in the experience
of conflict with the social environment for those in the minority group
(Lazarus & Folkman, 1984; Mirowsky & Ross, 1989; Pearlin, 1989).
Symbolic interaction and social comparison theories, for example, argue that the social environment organizes self-experience (Stryker &
Statham, 1985). Thus, negative regard from others leads to negative
self-regard (Rosenberg, 1979). In consequence, stigmatized individuals
develop both adaptive and maladaptive responses to the hostile social
environment that may include mental health concerns, self-hate, shy-
ness, and obsessive perseveration upon stigmatizing characteristics
(Meyer, 1995). At the center of these theoretical explanations is the ar-
ticulation of the incongruence between the minority person's culture,
needs and self-experience and the societal structures of his or her social
environment.

Allport (1954) describes vigilance as a particular trait that stigmatized individuals may develop to cope defensively with their minority
status. High levels of stigma would lead to hypervigilance–pervasive
expectations of rejection–of the minority components of their identity.
This hypervigilance, by definition, is chronic, and by implication, is
psychologically exhausting. Hetrick and Martin (1987) describe "learning to hide" as the most common coping strategy among gay adolescents, and this strategy is addressed frequently by other authors as well
(Cadwell, 1992; Cornett, 1993; Meyer, 1995). Similarly, Joachim and
Acorn (2000) review the theoretical literature on concealing one's status as chronically ill and find that these individuals experience a constant process of monitoring and evaluation related to disclosure in order

to avoid repetitive stigmatizing experiences. It follows, then, that high levels of perceived stigma for those who are gay and those who are chronically ill will lead to high levels of distress as they feel they must remain ever vigilant to avoid being harmed, psychologically or otherwise (Charmaz, 1991). Moreover, when the discrete burdens of stigma regarding sexual orientation and chronic illness must be contended with concurrently by the same individual, the demand for vigilance and the resulting level of minority stress may be overwhelming. The constant vigilance required for this type of chronic stigma management has negative implications not only for the development and maintenance of stable self-esteem, but also for successfully seeking out and receiving necessary medical care (Dean, 2000; Meyer, 1995).

COPING AND SOCIAL SUPPORT

What coping strategies might help gay men living with NHIVCIs to minimize the internalization of pejorative self-appraisals associated with a stigmatized identity? What combinations of information management techniques, interaction rituals, and internal definitions of self and others might allow these stigmatized individuals to maintain self-respect and deflect negative reactions and/or perceived negative reactions of others? How can these men be helped to buffer the persistent, multilevel assaults on the goodness of their identities within a social context that fails to reflect their specific illness experiences?

Social and psychological theories and research from diverse perspectives converge in agreement that accessing and receiving social support is a primary coping strategy for mitigating against isolation and stigmatization and promoting the development of a positive identity (Frable et al., 1998; Schreurs & deRidder, 1997). According to social identity, ego identity, and cultural conflict theories, developing a positive group identity will promote positive self-perceptions (Erikson, 1968; Porter & Washington, 1993; Tajfel, 1978). Similar others provide critical social comparison information for organizing one's self-concept and evaluating the self with respect to group membership. Thus, having both a positive gay identity and a positive identity as living with a chronic illness may be dependent, at least in part, upon the *perceived* availability of social supports. What one person sees as support, another may see as unhelpful (Schreurs & deRidder, 1997). The concept of perceived social support is therefore a significant one, as it captures the experiential, subjective perception of whether or not one has access to what he considers to be support.

Most gay men, whether living with an illness or not, are likely to perceive the availability of attuned social supports as limited (Ball, 1998). More often than not, this perception is likely to reflect an accurate assessment of one's social reality–even more so for gay men living with non-HIV chronic illnesses. While medical and psychosocial supports may exist for people living with chronic illnesses, they are not attuned to the role that sexual orientation plays in one's construction of his illness experience (with the important exception of HIV-related services). Likewise, while social supports exist for gay men to address their sexual identity, these supports are not attuned to issues of chronic illness (again with the exception of HIV-related supports). While social supports that speak to some parts of the self but not others can certainly be useful, stopgap measures, for example, a patient support group that does not attend to issues of sexual orientation, or a gay men's support group that does not explicitly address issues of chronic illness, the opportunity for locating a social space that promotes identity integration and offers affirmation of both of these fundamental aspects of identity *at the same time* is generally absent for this population.

GUIDELINES FOR SUPPORTING GAY MEN LIVING WITH NHIVCIs

Multiply stigmatized, physically ill, and socially invisible even within their own sexual minority group, gay men living with NHIVCIs present the social service provider with a complex array of psychosocial concerns. The provision of attuned services to this population calls for invoking a broad spectrum of roles and accompanying skills including clinical intervention, concrete service provision, and advocacy. Acknowledging a traumatic legacy of inaccurate pathologizing on the part of helping professionals related to both gay men and those living with a chronic illness, while mining current theory and practice principles related to other stigmatized groups, may help us to develop flexible and broadly applicable intervention strategies for intervening with this population across a wide range of modalities.

Recognizing the Legacy of Pathology

When working with gay men living with chronic illnesses, providers must be aware of the conscious and unconscious impact that the pathologizing by helping professionals, in particular, of both homosexuality and chronic illness has had on this population. In the domains of psychology and clinical social work, for example, psychoanalytic theory dominated clinical practice for the first half of the 20th century (Schoenberg & Goldberg, 1985). When little empirical evidence regarding bio-psychological development was available to the practitioner, theoretical assumptions about mysterious phenomena were not infrequently substituted for hard facts (Mitchell, 1981). These assumptions then provided practitioners with a definition of physical and psychological health and a road map for intervention where otherwise none would have existed. However, as subsequent theorists and researchers have pointed out, these practice principles were often more useful for binding the conscious and unconscious anxieties of practitioners than for helping those who sought out their services (Abelove, 1993; Frommer, 1995). Specific to this discussion, negative evaluations of homosexuality and physical illnesses as symptomatic of unresolved, deep psychological conflict often quelled medical and mental health providers' own psychological conflicts around not knowing as well as social anxieties related to difference, while doing damage to those in need of psychosocial support (Friedman & Downey, 1993).

Fortunately, subsequent advances in biology, descriptive psychiatry, the neural sciences, physiology, psychopharmacology, and clinical, developmental and neuropsychology have invalidated many of the pathology-based hypotheses regarding both sexual orientation and the psychosomatic attributions to genuine physical health concerns. While these advances bode well for current practice and future training of providers, it is important to recognize that the historically skeptical disposition of practitioners toward both gay and chronically ill clients continues to have a role in shaping a potential client's perceptions of the so-called "helping" professions. As a result, when a gay man requests medical or psychological help to address a chronic health concern, he may be likely to anticipate an overtly or, more probably, covertly hostile reception by his service provider. Therefore, creating an opportunity for compassionate engagement with gay men living with NHIVCIs may be a particularly delicate process. By directly addressing and normalizing the potential concerns of clients regarding prejudice, earned mistrust of healthcare professionals, and fear of stigmatization, a provider can take an essential first step toward offering a healing experience of empathic attunement (Cornett, 1993).

Promoting Empowerment

Social service providers working with gay men living with NHIVCIs must recognize the deleterious effects that the external environment can have on self-esteem and cohesive identity development. In response to external stressors, models of intervention need to stress the importance of self-esteem and identity cohesion (Garrett & Weissman, 2001; Kohut, 1984). Since alienation from both self and others is frequently part of the experience of living as both a gay man and as someone who is physically ill, practice must emphasize an integrative, biopsychosocial approach to intervention, with a keen eye on facilitating empowerment strategies for helping these men to proactively navigate their social environments.

A gay man has experienced dramatic external definition and moral judgment throughout his life (Cornett, 1993). Likewise, a person living with a chronic illness must deal with being devalued and marginalized (Joachim & Acorn, 2000). So, for a gay man living with NHIVCIs, it is crucial to provide opportunities in which he can experience a sense of expertise about defining *himself* rather than a replay of being defined by others. To this end, contemporary relational and intersubjective theories of clinical practice may provide useful resources for building strategies for intervention (Aron, 1996). Providers can forgo making expert interpretations and offering unsolicited advice, and instead privilege and work to amplify a client's narration of his experience. Facilitating a self-generated narrative serves to identify, clarify, coalesce, and organize what the client is communicating, rather than prioritize a provider's interpreting and ascribing either different or deeper meanings to a client's experience (Cornett, 1993; Kohut, 1977). Implicit in this strategy is the recognition that "expert"-based interpretations are biased social constructions, which for people who are gay and/or chronically ill, can lead to further stigmatization. Since the heterosexist, disease-phobic foundations of our culture unavoidably infiltrate any social service, a provider must continually guard against the tendency to offer unintentionally or unconsciously heterosexist and/or illness phobic, patient-blaming interventions. The overarching goal here is to differentiate this helping relationship from previous help-seeking experiences, which may have given life to, reinforced, and/or maintained expressions of self-criticism, self-loathing and shame.

Group Work with Gay Men Living with NHIVCIs

Since the psychosocial issues facing all gay men living with NHIVCIs are the result of adapting to an environment that has denied them both recognition and acceptance, psychosocial groups serving this population can provide a healing antidote to a history of isolation, deprivation and stigmatization related to this aspect of their psychosocial experience. Regardless of the particular focus of any group or its duration, opportunities for socialization with like others can promote the collaborative creation of effective coping strategies to offset self-perceptions of a devalued identity (Ball, 1996).

With the exception of services related to HIV, support groups for people living with chronic illnesses may have been sources of distress for gay men as they reinforced feelings of invisibility and shame within a presumed heterosexual context, rather than offering resources for affiliation and validation. Thus, gay men living with NHIVCIs may frequently enter a group with a legacy of psychological isolation surrounding their illness and may at first have difficulty relating openly to other men about this part of their lives (Ball, 1996; 1998). When a leader helps a group to recognize and employ their communal resources for support, members can begin to counteract their collective history of minority stress and disenfranchisement. Groups offer an opportunity to clarify emotional priorities and increase the capacity for building cohesive and responsive interpersonal networks that offer expansive, inclusive definitions of health, masculinity, attractiveness, self-worth and wellness that are less fettered by externally imposed limitations on these concepts (Ball & Lipton, 1996).

Responding to Ethnocultural Diversity

While the social service practice literature has begun to acknowledge the role of cultural competence in providing services to gay men in general, there remains a paucity of literature on culturally sensitive practice with gay men who are part of ethnocultural minorities (Adams & Kimmel, 1997; Colon, 2001; Crisp, 1998; Diaz, 1997; Fukuyama & Ferguson, 2000; Greene, 1996; Martinez & Sullivan, 1998; Rodriguez, 1996). The literature's biased focus on the experience of white, middle-class, younger, openly gay men suggests that neither theory nor research on this population is necessarily relevant to members of many of its subgroups. Instead, the marginalized place of ethnic and racial minorities as well older people within the literature on gay men parallels the social realities of minority populations within both society at large and the gay community (Greene, 1996). Clearly, being gay does not preclude one from experiencing or fomenting ethnocultural prejudice (Fukuyama & Ferguson, 2000). Thus, it is imperative for providers to recognize the additional stigmas of discrimination based upon race, ethnicity, and age with which some men living with NHIVCIs must also contend, and to assess how these additional cultural factors affect these clients' psychosocial stressors and coping opportunities.

In both individual and group modalities, interventions must help gay men living with NHIVCIs to articulate and validate their particular ethnocultural experiences and conflicts in relation to both sexual orientation and living with a chronic illness. For example, African-American gay men may experience identity conflicts as they search for an affirming space amid three problematic environments: their African-American heritage that may have homo-negative aspects; the hegemonic, racist white gay culture; and the historically racist, culturally insensitive, heterosexist health care system (Adams & Kimmel, 1997; Crisp, 1998; Greene, 1996; Martinez & Sullivan, 2000). Several authors explore similar difficulties that arise from the interplay of race, ethnicity and sexual orientation for Latino and Asian-American gay men (Colon, 2001; Diaz, 1997; Pares-Avila, 1994; Rodriguez, 1996). A service provider who actively works to educate him/herself about the ethnocultural concerns of a client can strive to provide a safe, attuned space for ventilating painful feelings of alienation from multiple out-groups, strengthening self-esteem, and developing effective coping strategies for traversing seemingly exclusive cultural groups. The converse also is true. A practitioner who ignores or obviates the significance of cultural competency risks reinforcing traumatic experiences of neglect and marginalization–and endangering the health of minority clients (Dean, 2000)

Addressing Aging

In addition to ethnocultural factors, age also impacts on one's identity as a gay man and as a healthy, vital individual. Since the devastation of a generation of gay men by AIDS, the concept of longevity for gay men has undergone radical redefinition (Ball, 1998; Rofes, 1996). Men in their 40s and 50s join those in their 60s, 70s, and 80s in the developmental task of survivorship as they work through loss and strive for regeneration. In tackling these difficult tasks, middle-aged and older gay men find that they must construct an identity outside of the mainstream gay culture that lauds youth and pays little regard to the realities of aging, including onset of chronic illness and disability (Adams & Kimmel, 1997). The current generation of older gay men, the first to have had the possibility of living as openly gay for the duration of their adult lives, demonstrates an impressive resilience in the face of ostracism, stigma, and invisibility. Supporting such strengths requires a provider to carefully assess the impact of aging on a client's self-concept and its relevance to capacities for coping with chronic illness.

Advocating for Change

Advocacy is an integral part of any social service provider's repertoire of interventions and is inevitably necessary when working with marginalized, underserved populations such as gay men living with NHIVCIs. Homophobia and heterosexism in medical practice are realities. A recent survey of nursing students showed that 8-12% "despised" lesbian, gay and bisexual people, 5-12% found them "disgusting," and 43% thought gay and bisexual people should keep their sexuality private (Kaiser Permanente National Diversity Council, 1998). Another study revealed that more than 20% of male physicians in cities with populations between 25,000 and 50,000 people could be described as homophobic (Telex, 1999). Because the current social environment in general, and health care system in particular, are rarely patient friendly or responsive to the needs of sexual minorities, advocacy on behalf of gay men living with NHIVCIs must follow several avenues simultaneously. On the macro level, a provider can employ social activism toward changing public policy to provide: equal rights to gay men; universal access to affordable, comprehensive health care; and medical and ancillary treatment that is informed by awareness and acceptance of the impact of sexual orientation on health issues. On the micro level, these goals translate into promoting access for clients to concrete services such as medical care, financial entitlements, and ancillary supports; advocating for patients' rights within specific health care settings; facilitating client self-determination and empowerment in the face of paternalistic health care systems; and educating service providers about the specific psychosocial needs of gay men living with NHIVCIs.

Social service providers can advocate for specific steps to create environments in health care settings and patient care organizations that are welcoming to gay-identified patients. Posting nondiscrimination statements inclusive of sexual orientation, displaying posters or pamphlets with gay friendly, gay positive messages, subscribing to gay-oriented news or entertainment periodicals, acknowledging important days of observance such as Gay Pride, and recognizing domestic partnerships and other nontraditional family relationships all convey to a potential gay client that they will be safe and respected (GLMA, 1999). Likewise, in-service trainings that address the unique psychosocial stressors of gay men living with NHIVCIs can increase provider awareness and stimulate proactive efforts to outreach to these men and respond with culturally competent medical and social services.

CONCLUSION

The opportunity to explore the concerns of gay men living with chronic illnesses *other* than HIV might never have been possible without the radical ways in which advocates for people living with HIV have propelled the demand for equal rights for gay people to a front burner issue in our culture at large, and particularly within the arena of health care (Kramer, 1997; Rofes, 1996). As the recognition by medical and social service providers that HIV is a persistent reality rather than a short-term crisis is now being operationalized in programs and policies, the time is ripe to build on the lessons of empowerment from the legacy of HIV. These models of activism and service provision can be joined with those of organizations that target many other chronic illnesses that also affect gay men, but whose services have not considered the specific impact of sexual orientation on the experience of living with a chronic illness.

Advocacy efforts on behalf of gay men living with NHIVCIs require a dual focus of attention: heterosexually oriented medical and patient advocacy organizations on the one hand, and gay identified medical and social service organizations on the other. While the focus of advocacy with the former is on increasing cultural competence with gay men, the focus with the latter must be on increasing awareness of the breadth of health care concerns that gay men experience. These serious health concerns are much broader than those related to HIV and other sexually transmitted diseases which gay identified health organizations have traditionally addressed. If we can harness the synergistic effects of attuned social service provision to broad ranging advocacy interventions that foster empowerment and visibility, then social service providers can begin to develop a more comprehensive, inclusive medical and social service delivery system that addresses the particular impact of sexual orientation on living with a broad range of life-challenging illnesses.

REFERENCES

Aron, L. (1996). *A meeting of minds: Mutuality in psychoanalysis.* Hillsdale, NJ: The Analytic Press, Inc.

Abelove, H. (1993). Freud, male homosexuality and the Americans. In H. Abelove (Ed.), *The lesbian and gay studies reader* (pp. 381-393). New York: Routledge.

Adams, C.L., & Kimmel, D.C. (1997). Exploring the lives of older African American gay men. In B. Greene (Ed.), *Ethnic and cultural diversity among lesbians and gay men: Psychological perspectives on lesbian and gay issues, Vol. 3* (pp.132-151). Thousand Oaks, CA: Sage Publications.

Allport, G.W. (1954). *The nature of prejudice.* Reading, MA: Addison-Wesley.

Ball, S. (Ed.). (1998). *The HIV negative gay man.* Harrington Park Press: New York.

Ball, S., & Lipton, B. (1996). Group work with gay men. In G.L. Greif & P.H. Ephross (Eds.), *Group work with populations at risk* (pp. 165-182). New York: Oxford Press.

Brooks, V.R. (1981). *Minority stress and lesbian women.* Lexington, MA: Lexington Books, D.C. Heath & Co.

Cadwell, S. (1992). Twice removed: The stigma suffered by gay men with AIDS. *Smith Studies in Social Work, 61*(3), 236-246.

Center for Disease Control (2002). *HIV/AIDS surveillance report, Vol. 13(2).* Retrieved September 15, 2002, from http://www.cdc.gov/hiv/stats/hasr1302/table10.htm

Charmaz, K. (1991). *Good day, bad days: The self in control, illness and time.* New Brunswick, NJ: Rutgers University Press.

Chauncey, G. (1994). *Gay New York: Gender, urban culture, and the making of the gay male world 1890-1940.* New York: Basic Books.

Colon, E. (2001). An ethnographic study of six Latino men. *Journal of Gay and Lesbian Social Services, 12*(3-4), 77-92.

Conlin, D., & Smith, J. (1985). *Group psychotherapy for gay men.* In J. Gonsiorek (Ed.), *Homosexuality and psychotherapy: A practitioner's handbook of affirmative models* (pp.105-112). New York: The Haworth Press, Inc.

Cornett, C. (Ed.) (1993). *Affirmative dynamic psychotherapy with gay men.* Northvale, NJ: Jason Aronson, Inc.

Crisp, D. (1998). African American gay men: Developmental issues, choices and self-concept. *Family Therapy, 25*(3): 161-168.

Cuijpers, P. (1998). Prevention of depression in chronic general medical disorders: A pilot study. *Psychological Reports, 82,* 735-738.

Dean, L. (2000). Lesbian, gay, bisexual, and transgender health: Findings and concerns. *Journal of the Gay and Lesbian Medical Association, 4*(3), 101-151.

Diaz, R. (1997). Latino gay men and psycho-cultural barriers to HIV prevention. In M. Levine and P. Nardi (Eds.), *In changing times: Gay men and lesbians encounter HIV/AIDS* (pp. 221-244). Chicago: University of Chicago Press.

Donoghue, P., & Siegel, M. (2001). *Sick and tired of feeling sick and tired* (2nd ed.). New York: W.W. Norton & Company.

Erikson, E. (1950). *Childhood and society.* New York: W.W. Norton.

Frable, D.E.S., Platt, L., & Hoey, S. (1998). Concealable stigma and positive self-perceptions: Feeling better around similar others. *Journal of Personality and Social Psychology, 24*(4), 909-922.

Frable, D.E.S., Wortman, C., & Joseph, J. (1997). Predicting self-esteem, well-being, and distress in a cohort of gay men: The importance of cultural stigma, personal visibility, community networks, and positive identity. *Journal of Personality, 65*(3), 599-624.

Friedman, R.C., & Downey, J. (1993). Psychoanalysis, psychobiology and homosexuality. *Journal of the American Psychoanalytic Association, 41*(4), 1159-1198.

Frommer, M.S. (1995). Homosexuality and psychoanalysis: Technical considerations revisited. *Psychoanalytic Dialogues, 4.*

Fukuyama, M.A., & Ferguson, A.D. (2000). Lesbian, gay and bisexual people of color: Understanding cultural complexity and managing multiple oppressions. In R. Perez & K. DeBord (Eds.), *Handbook of counseling and psychotherapy with lesbian, bay and bisexual clients* (pp. 81-105). Washington, DC: American Psychological Association.

Garrett, C. & Weisman, M.G. (2001). A self-psychological perspective on chronic illness. *Clinical Social Work Journal, 29*(2), 119-132.

Gay & Lesbian Medical Association. (1994). *Anti-gay discrimination in medicine: Results of a national survey of lesbian, gay, and bisexual physicians.* San Francisco, CA: Author.

Gay & Lesbian Medical Association. (1999). *Mission statement.* Retrieved on July 12, 2002, from http://www.glma.org/home

Gay and Lesbian Medical Association & Columbia Center for Gay, Lesbian, Bisexual and Transgender Health (2000). *The GLMA-Columbia University white paper on GLBT health.* San Francisco, CA: Author.

Gay & Lesbian Medical Association (2001). *Lesbian, gay, bisexual and transgender companion document to healthy people 2010.* San Francisco, CA: Author.

Goffman, E. (1963). *Stigma: Notes on the management of a spoiled identity.* Englewood Cliffs, NJ: Prentice-Hall.

Goin, M.K. (1990). Emotional survival and the aging body. In R.A. Nemiroff & C.A. Colarusso (Eds.), *New dimensions in adult development* (pp.518-531). New York: Basic Books, Inc.

Goodheart, C.D., & Lansing, M.H. (1996). *Treating people with chronic disease: A psychological guide.* Washington, D.C.: American Psychological Association.

Greene, B. (1996). Lesbian and gay men of color: The legacy of ethnosexual mythologies in heterosexism and homophobia. In E.D. Rothblum & L.A. Bond (Eds.), *Preventing heterosexism and homophobia: Primary prevention of psychopathology* (pp. 59-70). Thousand Oaks, CA: Sage Publications.

Herdt, G., Beeler, J., and Rawls, T.W. (1997). Life course diversity among old lesbians and gay men: A study in Chicago. *Journal of Gay, Lesbian and Bisexual Identity, 2*(3/4), 231-246.

Herek, G.M. (1990). Illness, stigma and AIDS. In P.T. Costa and G.R. VandenBos (Eds), *Psychological aspects of serious illness: Chronic conditions, fatal diseases, and clinical care* (pp. 107-149). Washington, DC: American Psychological Association.

Hetrick, E.S., & Martin, A.D. (1984). Ego-dystonic homosexuality: A developmental view. In E.S. Hetrick & T.S. Stein (Eds.), *Innovations in psychotherapy with homosexuals* (pp. 2-21). Washington, DC: American Psychiatric Association Press.

Joachim, G., & Acorn, S. (2000). Stigma of visible and invisible chronic conditions. *Journal of Advanced Nursing, 32*(1), 243-248.

Jones, E., Farina, A., Hastorf, A., Markus, H., Miller, D., & Scott, R. (1984). *Social stigma: The psychology of marked relationships.* New York: Freeman.

Kaiser Permanente National Diversity Council & Kaiser Permanente National Diversity Department (1998). *A provider's handbook on culturally competent care: Lesbian, gay, bisexual and transgendered population.* Los Angeles, CA: Kaiser Permanente.

Katz, A., & Martin, K. (1982). *A handbook of services for the handicapped.* Westport: CT: Greenwood Press.

Katz, I. (1981). *Stigma: A social psychological analysis.* Hillsdale, NJ: Erlbaum.

Kohut, H. (1984). *How does analysis cure?* Chicago: The University of Chicago Press.

Krajeski, J.P. (1986). Psychotherapy with gay men and lesbians: A history of controversy. In T.S. Stein & C.J. Cohen (Eds.), *Contemporary perspectives on psychotherapy with lesbians and gay men* (pp. 9-25). New York: Plenum.

Kramer, L. (1997). *Reports from the Holocaust: The story of an AIDS activist.* New York: St. Martin's Press.

Landis, B.J. (1991). Uncertainty, spiritual well-being, and psychosocial adjustment to chronic illness. *Dissertation Abstracts International, 52*(08), 4124B (University Microfilms No. AA19200662).

LaPlante, M. P., & Carlson, D. (1996). *Disability in the United States: Prevalence and causes, 1992* (Disability Statistics Report No. 6). Washington, DC: National Institute on Disability and Rehabilitation Research.

Laumann, O., Gangnon, J.H., Michael, R.T., & Michael, S. (1994). *The social organization of sexuality: Sexual practices in the United States.* Chicago: University of Chicago Press.

Lazarus, R.S., & Folkman, S. (1984). *Stress, appraisal and coping.* New York: Springer Publishing Company.

Lewis, J. (1999). Status passages: The experience of HIV-positive gay men. *Journal of Homosexuality, 37*(3), 87-115.

Lipton, B. (1998). The psychosocial impact of colon and rectal disease on gay men. *Seminars in Colon and Rectal Surgery, 9*(2), 149-154.

Lipton, B. (1997). Responding to non-HIV invisible chronic illness within the gay male community. *Journal of Gay and Lesbian Social Services 7*(1), 93-98.

Martin, J., & Hunter, S. (2001). *Lesbian, gay, bisexual and transgender issues in social work: A comprehensive bibliography with annotations.* Alexandria, VA: Council on Social Work Education.

Martinez, D.G., & Sullivan, S.C. (2000). African American gay men and lesbians: Examining the complexity of gay identity development. In L.A. Letha (Ed.), *Human behavior in the social environment from an African American perspective* (pp. 243-264). Athens, GA: University of Georgia Press.

Meyer, I.H. (1995). Minority stress and mental health in gay men. *Journal of Health and Social Behavior, 36*, 38-56.

Mirowsky, J., & Ross, C. (1980). Minority status, ethnic culture, and distress: A comparison of Black, Whites, Mexicans, and Mexican Americans. *American Journal of Sociology, 86*, 479-95.

Mitchell, S. (1978). Psychodynamics, homosexuality and the question of pathology. *Psychiatry, 41*, 254-263.

Paradis, B.A. (1993). A self-psychological approach to the treatment of gay men with AIDS. *Clinical Social Work Journal, 21*(4), 405-416.

Pares-Avila (1994). Issues in the psychosocial care of Latino gay men with HIV infection. In S. Cadwell & R. Burnham, Jr. (Eds.), *Therapists on the front line: Psychotherapy with gay men in the age of AIDS* (pp. 339-362). Washington, DC: American Psychiatric Press.

Pearlin, L.I. (1982). The social context of stress. In L. Goldberger & S. Breznitz (Eds.), *Handbook of stress: Theoretical and clinical aspects* (pp. 367-379). New York: Academic Press.

Phillips, M.J. (1990). Damaged goods: Oral narrative of the experience of a disability in American culture. *Social Science and Medicine, 30, 849-857.*

Porter, J., & Washington, R. (1993). Minority identity and self-esteem. In J. Blake & J. Hagen (Eds.), *Annual review of sociology* (pp. 139-161). Palo Alto, CA: Annual Reviews.

Rodriguez, R. (1996). Clinical issues in identity development in gay Latino men. In C. Alexander (Ed.), *Gay and lesbian mental health: A sourcebook for practitioners* (pp. 127-157). New York: Haworth Park Press.

Rofes, E. (1996). *Reviving the tribe: Regenerating gay men's sexuality and culture in the ongoing epidemic.* New York: Harrington Park Press.

Rosenberg, M. (1979). *Conceiving the self.* New York: Basic Books.

Rosenfeld, D. (1999). Identity work among the homosexual elderly. *Journal of Aging Studies, 13*(2), 121.

Sadownick, D. (1996). *Sex between men.* San Francisco, CA: Harper San Francisco

Sears, J.T., & Williams, W.L (Eds.) (1997). *Overcoming heterosexism and homophobia: Strategies that work.* New York: Columbia University Press.

Schoenberg, R., & Goldberg, R.S. (Eds.) (1985). *With compassion towards some: Homosexuality and social work in America.* New York: Harrington Park Press.

Schreurs, K., & de Ridder, T. (1997). Integration of coping and social support perspectives: Implications for the study of adaptation to chronic diseases. *Clinical Psychology Review, 17*(1), 89-112.

Shuman, R. (1996). *The psychology of chronic illness.* New York: Basic Books.

Signorile, M. (1997). *Life outside: The Signorile report on gay men: Sex, drugs, muscles, and the passage of life.* New York: Harper Collins Publishers.

Sontag, S. (1978). *Illness as metaphor.* New York: Farrar, Straus & Giroux.

Sontag, S. (1988). *AIDS and its metaphors.* New York: Farrar, Straus & Giroux.

Stryker, S., & Statham, A. (1985). Symbolic interaction and role theory. In G. Lindzey & E. Aronson (Eds.), *Handbook of social psychology* (pp. 311-378). New York: Random House.

Tajfel, H. (1978). *The social psychology of minorities* (Report No. 38). London: Minority Rights Group.

Telex, C. (1999). Attitudes of physicians in New Mexico toward gay men and lesbians. *Journal of the Gay and Lesbian Medical Association, 3*(3), pp. 121-130.

Thorne, S.E. (1993). *Negotiating health care: The social context of chronic illness.* Newbury Park, CA: Sage.

U.S. Census Bureau. (2002). *Resident population estimates of the United States by age and sex: April 1, 1990 to July 1, 1999, with short-term projection to November 1, 2000* [Data file]. Available from U.S. Census Bureau Website, http://eire.census.gov/popest/archives/national/nation2/intfile2-1.txt

Gay Men Living with Chronic Illness or Disability: A Sociocultural, Minority Group Perspective on Mental Health

William F. Hanjorgiris
Joseph F. Rath
John H. O'Neill

SUMMARY. This paper examines the experiences of gay men living with disabilities or chronic illness from a social constructivist perspective. Emphasizing the sociocultural aspects of disability, such an approach recognizes that the questions asked and the answers given about disability are embedded in sociohistorical contexts, and that language both shapes and reveals underlying assumptions and behaviors related to disability. Using Kameny's (1971) concept of sociological minority, it is proposed that gay men and persons with disabilities constitute minority groups with experi-

---

William F. Hanjorgiris, PhD, maintains a private psychotherapy practice in NYC and can be reached at 380 Second Avenue, Suite 302, New York, NY 10010.

Joseph F. Rath, PhD, is a research scientist, Rusk Institute of Rehabilitation Medicine, New York University School of Medicine, 400 East 34th Street, New York, NY 10016.

John H. O'Neill, PhD, CRC, is Professor and Coordinator, Counselor Education, Department of Educational Foundations and Counseling Programs, Hunter College, City University of New York, 695 Park Avenue, New York, NY 10021.

[Haworth co-indexing entry note]: "Gay Men Living with Chronic Illness or Disability: A Sociocultural, Minority Group Perspective on Mental Health." Hanjorgiris, William F., Joseph F. Rath, and John H. O'Neill. Co-published simultaneously in *Journal of Gay & Lesbian Social Services* (Harrington Park Press, an imprint of The Haworth Press, Inc.) Vol. 17, No. 2, 2004, pp. 25-41; and: *Gay Men Living with Chronic Illnesses and Disabilities: From Crisis to Crossroads* (ed: Benjamin Lipton) Harrington Park Press, an imprint of The Haworth Press, Inc., 2004, pp. 25-41. Single or multiple copies of this article are available for a fee from The Haworth Document Delivery Service [1-800-HAWORTH, 9:00 a.m. - 5:00 p.m. (EST). E-mail address: docdelivery@haworthpress.com].

http://www.haworthpress.com/web/JGLSS
Digital Object Identifier: 10.1300/J041v17n02_02

ences in common with those of other recognized minority groups. Implications for mental health practitioners providing services to gay men with disabilities are addressed. *[Article copies available for a fee from The Haworth Document Delivery Service: 1-800-HAWORTH. E-mail address: <docdelivery@haworthpress.com> Website: <http://www.HaworthPress.com> © 2004 by The Haworth Press, Inc. All rights reserved.]*

KEYWORDS. Counseling/psychotherapy, chronic illness, disability, discrimination, minority groups, gay males, identity development, mental health, social constructivism

As the U.S. population ages, gay men, like members of the general population, are likely to develop at least one chronic illness or disability in their lifetime (LaPlante & Carlson, 1996). Regrettably, mental health training programs, with few exceptions, do not adequately address the unique concerns of gay men or persons with disabilities independently, let alone in tandem. Resources have been created to assist mental health practitioners in providing services to gay men (e.g., American Psychological Association, 2000; Bohan, 1996; Campos & Goldfried, 2001; Davies & Neal, 1996; Haldeman, 2001; Perez, DeBord, & Bieschke, 2000), as well as to individuals with disabilities (Marinelli & Dell Orto, 1999; Olkin, 2001; Phelps, 1998; Purnell & Paulanka, 1998). Recently, scholars and researchers have begun to acknowledge the challenges that confront gay men living with disabilities (Atkins & Marston, 1999; O'Neill & Hird, 2001). Yet no resource currently exists that comprehensively addresses the psychosocial needs of gay men living with chronic illness or disability.

In this chapter, we will propose an avenue for scholarly inquiry that draws parallels between the experiences of persons with disabilities, gay men, and members of racial/ethnic minority groups (cf. Corbett, 1994; Gordon & Rosenblum, 2001). Rather than using a traditional essentialist/biomedical approach, the authors will emphasize sociocultural aspects of being designated "different" by taking a social constructivist approach to understanding chronic illness and disability. We will articulate how language shapes and reveals underlying assumptions and informs overt behavior related to the understanding of disability and gay identity. Finally, an effort will be made to extrapolate from concepts created for other minority groups and apply the extant theory, paradigms, and heuristics to providing mental health services to gay men with chronic illness or disability.

SOCIOLOGICAL MINORITIES

Power, voice, status, agency, and choice are privileges taken for granted by majority individuals but often denied to minorities in American society. Compounding this injustice is confusion regarding the socio-legal intent of the term "minority." According to Kameny's (1971) concept of "sociological minority," a minority group is defined by the following criteria: group members (a) share a minority characteristic, (b) deal with discrimination and prejudice, (c) are depersonalized and not judged on their own merits, and (d) internalize a "we-they" mentality. Using this definition, both people with disabilities and gay men can be understood as comprising minority groups. People with disabilities and gay men, like all minority groups, cannot escape being defined by their social group memberships (Adams, Bell, & Griffin, 1997). Their lives include routine exposure to the stress of negative attitudes, discrimination, oppression, and prejudice (Lewis, Derlega, Berndt, Morris, & Rose, 2001; Livneh, 1991b; Simon, 1998).

Although it generally can be stated that most people identified as being "different" have been impacted by prejudice, discrimination, negative bias, or oppression, each person's response to these stressors may differ based upon a myriad of factors (i.e., socioeconomic status, availability of community and family support systems, constitutional factors, and educational opportunity). The experience of gay men and people with disabilities differs from that of other minority groups in that members of these marginalized populations rarely have family members, neighbors, or important figures in the community who share their minority characteristic and can validate their experiences, offer advice, or serve as role models. As Longmore (1995) aptly noted:

> Not having a similarly identified family to belong to, it is difficult to develop a shared experience with family and community members. Common cultural experiences bind persons in each of society's minorities. When we are with disabled peers and share our stories, a common thread of survival, restricted choices, enforced poverty, and benign oppression is found in all of them. Consequently, there is power in difference and strength within the stories. (p. 11)

As increasing numbers of people with disabilities identify as members of a sociological minority group (Fine & Asch, 2000), disability activists have been able to advocate successfully for community rights and the opportunity for those who are disabled to gain control over their personal lives. Although a similar movement occurred within the gay community after the 1969 Stonewall rebellion, gay men have yet to achieve the civil rights and liberties allowed other minority groups in America. The advent of the AIDS crisis forced gay men to divert energy from the pursuit of equal rights to fighting for access to adequate medical care and treatment. Today, compassionate care may be provided to gay men with AIDS; yet acceptance, equal rights, and economic opportunity continue to elude most gay people. As members of a community already struggling to cope with the stress of discrimination (DiPlacido, 1998), gay men who develop a chronic illness or disability (or people with disabilities who come out as gay) may find themselves overwhelmed and especially vulnerable to adjustment problems.

Gay men with disabilities who are from racial/ethnic minority backgrounds may face multiple sources of discrimination based on sexual orientation, disability, and race/ethnicity, resulting in a kind of double or triple jeopardy (cf. O'Neill & Hird, 2001). The relative salience of any one minority characteristic or identity will vary from person to person, time to time, and place to place depending on social context. An individual's ability to "pass" as a member of the majority is also a factor. Discrimination may also come from within the gay community, as mirrored by a gay media that extols the virtues of youth, physical ability and attractiveness. A typical personal ad on a popular gay Website reflects these biases (e.g., ableism, ageism, and lookism):

> VGL masc, musc, 30-something guy, sensitive and intelligent, gym tight body seeking same for LTR or good times. I keep myself in shape by hitting the gym 3-5X/week. Not interested in guys without pics–hey, it's only fair I showed you mine. NO FATS, FEMS, guys with baggage or guys on Prozac! I am DISEASE FREE UB2. Sorry if this sounds harsh guys just being honest. It's all about chemistry right?! Prefer dudes my age or younger. Give me a shout.

Whatever the source(s) of discrimination, mental health professionals need to be aware of the negative sequelae of discrimination and the problems in living that result when one is designated as "different" from mainstream society. In particular, while ableism, ageism, and lookism abound in both straight and gay personal ads, the pejorative reference to those who are "diseased" seems specific to gay ads and reflects the prominence of this particular stigma among many gay men.

HEALTHY MINORITY IDENTITY DEVELOPMENT

"People who have been socialized in an oppressive environment, and who accept the dominant groups' ideology about their group, have learned to accept a definition of themselves that is hurtful and limiting" (Adams et al., 1997, p. 21). As the example of the personal ad above illustrates, members of oppressed groups may, paradoxically, exhibit the same prejudicial attitudes that they themselves have been forced to endure. For healthy identity development, gay men and persons with disabilities, like all minority group members, must undergo an identity development process that permits self-acceptance and allows the person to integrate identified differences into the self-concept.

Historically, services offered to people with disabilities focused primarily on personal acceptance of loss. Vash (1981) proposed an innovative three-stage identity development process for persons with disabilities that goes beyond a focus on acceptance of disability. In Stage 1, disability is seen as a tragedy. During Stage 2, disability is viewed as an inconvenience that can be mastered. At Stage 3, disability is seen as having contributed to the individual's growth as a person. Notably, Stage 3 recognizes that acceptance of disability may go beyond acceptance of loss.

Gill (1997) expanded the discourse to the group level and articulated stages of disability identity development that include (a) coming to feel one belongs (integrating into society), (b) coming home (integrating with the disability community), (c) coming together (internally integrating one's sameness and "different-ness"), and (d) coming out (integrating how one feels with how one presents to others). Similar developmental models also have been created to describe the process through which an individual develops a healthy gay, lesbian, or bisexual identity (see Bohan, 1996; D'Augelli, & Patterson, 2001; Gonsiorek & Weinrich, 1991), as well as to describe the development of racial/ethnic identities (see Atkinson & Hackett, 1998; Atkinson, Morten, & Sue, 1998).

Consistent with the theoretical conceptualizations of Vash (1981) and Gill (1997), Grant (1996) investigated the development of a "disability identity." Based upon the Minority Identity Development model of Atkinson et al. (1993), Grant developed and validated the Disability Identity Attitude Scale (DIAS). The DIAS documents the existence of four distinct phases of disability identity: (1) Dissociation, (2) Diffusion/Dysphoria, (3) Immersion/Solidarity, and (4) Introspective Acceptance. According to Grant, during Phase I (Dissociation), people with disabilities protect their self-identity by not associating with others who have disabilities. The avoidance may be based on negative attitudes toward the disabled population in general, discomfort regarding these negative thoughts, or negative contact with others regarding disability issues. In Phase 2 (Diffusion/Dysphoria), people with disabilities can experience considerable emotional distress and maintain self-identity by using certain defense mechanisms (e.g., projection, denial, displacement, and identification with the oppressor). In Phase 3 (Immersion/Solidarity), persons with disabilities begin to resolve their identity conflict by trying to understand and bond with the disability community/culture and distancing themselves from the dominant nondisabled community. Finally, in Phase 4 (Introspective Acceptance), individuals with disabilities can integrate positive and negative experiences with both the disabled and nondisabled communities and make reality-based judgments regarding their relationships to others in the disabled community and the nondisabled community.

Just as racial categories can be understood as social constructions (see, e.g., Graves, 2001), the designation of who is gay/straight or disabled/nondisabled depends greatly on context. For example, many people around the world engage in same-sex sexual behavior yet do not identify as lesbian, gay, or bisexual and are not identified as such by others (Herdt, 1997). The distinction among the concepts of sexual orientation, sexual behavior, and sexual identity has helped to explain why same-sex sexual activity does not always lead to a self-definition as gay or bisexual. Similarly, many persons with chronic conditions and/or functional limitations may not identify as having a disability and may not be identified as such by others.

Most Americans are unfamiliar with the specifics of the Americans with Disabilities Act (ADA, 1991) and are uncertain as to who can be considered "officially" disabled. For many, the term "disability" brings to mind a picture of a person in a wheelchair (O'Keefe, 1993), as depicted in the international symbol for disability. However, although mobility impairments may be the most easily recognizable of disabilities, not all disabilities result in the need for a wheelchair. The majority of people with disabilities do not have mobility impairments, and not all mobility impairments are chronic. Individuals may identify with a variety of illnesses and impairments yet may not use the term disability when describing themselves or their experiences.

In defining disability, the drafters of the ADA recognized the contextualized nature of disability and created a broad scope of situations under which an individual could benefit from its provisions (see Henderson & Bryan, 1997; Linton, 1998). Although recent court decisions have begun to impose limitations on the original spirit and intent of the ADA, individuals may be considered to have a disability if they have an impairment that creates a functional limitation in a major life activity (e.g., reading, learning, working, traveling, walking, etc.). Such a definition stems from the essentialist approach to understanding disability (i.e., one that understands disability as a limitation situated within the person).

However, the drafters of the ADA also recognized that disability and its associated discrimination is often "in the eye of the beholder," an approach consistent with a social constructivist perspective. Therefore, people with a history of a disability (e.g., cancer, substance abuse, etc.) or people perceived to have a disability (e.g., facial scaring from burns, obesity, etc.) are also covered by the ADA. The ADA even recognizes that discrimination related to disability can spread to those around the person with a disability. Consequently, those associated with a person who has a disability (e.g., the spouse of a person with HIV) are also protected against discrimination by the ADA.

DEFINING THE POPULATIONS:
A SOCIAL-CONSTRUCTIVIST APPROACH

A social constructivist approach recognizes that language both shapes and reveals underlying assumptions and overt behaviors related to disability. In other words, "our understandings are shaped by the language we employ and the categories we create to define and describe the phenomena we take to be reality" (Bohan & Russell, 1999, p. 15). From this perspective, limitations related to chronic illness/disability and sexual orientation are seen as located in the surroundings encountered (i.e., environments, social context, etc.) and the language used, rather than within the individual.

For social constructivists, the limitations that people with chronic illnesses/disabilities experience are not primarily due to their physical, mental, or emotional characteristics, but rather stem from the barriers created by the reactions and sociopolitical structure of the surrounding society (Linton, Mello, & O'Neill, 1996). For example, most people with chronic illness are eager to work and to interact socially with peers, but frequently are unable to do so because of the parentalistic and negative treatment encountered by employers, colleagues, peers, and others. Thus, many competent people with disabilities may be un/underemployed due to the various social, environmental, architectural, legal, religious, and political barriers to their career development. This situation may be expected to be compounded when the person with a chronic illness or disability is also gay.

This conceptualization stands in marked contrast to the prevailing ahistorical, universal essentialist approach that situates disability, disease, and sexual orientation as characteristics inherent in the individual (Bohan & Russell, 1999; Linton et al., 1996). Here, the use of the term "normal" (and by implication "abnormal") takes communication to a level of abstraction that allows for vagueness and ambiguity. When this occurs, there is seldom an opportunity to discuss the concrete, specific ways that individuals or groups differ. In such interactions, there is an assumed agreement between speaker and listener regarding what is normal that creates a sense of empathy or "us-ness." This process ". . . enhances social unity among those who feel they are normal" (Freilich, Raybeck, & Savishinsky, 1991, p. 22) and excludes the "other," or abnormal. It is more precise and meaningful to discuss specific differences between people, instead of evaluating whether those differences are normal or abnormal.

As the current paradigm of disability moves from a medical model (essentialist) to a minority-group model (social constructivist), the language used to describe disability has begun to change. The new language conveys different meanings and shifts the meta-communications into the sociopolitical realm (Linton et al., 1996). Much of the old language of disability could be considered "ableist" (i.e., parallel to terminology that is now recognized as racist or sexist). Some ableist language infers that people with disabilities are more childlike, dependent, passive, and incompetent than those without disabilities (e.g. "that poor, suffering soul"). Conversely, other ableist language can attribute unusual sensitivity, courage, or ability to people just because they have a disability (e.g., "a remarkable achievement for a person with a disability").

An important distinction exists between disability and handicap, even though the two terms often are used interchangeably. Disability refers to a functional limitation, condition, or physical impairment that is evident in the way a person looks, perceives the world, feels, moves, communicates, sees, hears, or processes information (World Health Organization, 1993). The disability can be visible or invisible, and it exists as a relatively permanent characteristic of the individual that does not vary from one context to another. In contrast, handicap is the limitation experienced by an individual in certain activities or environments, and the degree of handicap is relative to the situation. Handicap emerges as the person with a disability interacts with environments that do not accommodate that characteristic of the person. Thus, a handicap is not a characteristic of the individual, but arises from the environment. For example, people who use wheelchairs are not *handicapped*, but inaccessible buildings *handi-*

cap people who use wheelchairs. The distinction between disability and handicap emphasizes that a disability is not equally limiting in all situations and that society determines the degree of limitation imposed.

BEST PRACTICES IN MENTAL HEALTH

Mental health practitioners sometimes display paternalistic attitudes and expect clients with disabilities to yield to the advice and instructions they offer. When clients refuse to comply, clinicians may inappropriately label the behavior (e.g., denial, treatment resistance, acting out, personality disordered) rather than recognizing that their interventions may be incompatible with the clients' needs or desires. Thus, mental health practitioners need to examine personal knowledge, attitudes, and beliefs before they can begin to work effectively with clients who do not share their worldview (see Sue, Arrendondo, & McDavis, 1992).

If mental health providers have not made the effort to understand their individual feelings, beliefs, and attitudes regarding "difference," they may become part of an oppressive culture within the consulting room that mirrors the oppression experienced outside of it (Reeve, 2000). It is not surprising that clinicians may emulate majority cultural norms for functioning, which include good hearing and vision, physical independence and mobility, mental alertness, the ability to communicate primarily through the written and spoken word, and physical attractiveness. Such bias and countertransference reactions can present serious impediments to case conceptualization, treatment planning, and choice of intervention strategies.

Kemp and Mallinckrodt (1996) describe two fundamental errors made by mental health providers that negatively impact upon case conceptualization. The first type of error, an error of omission, occurs when the clinician fails to ask about critical aspects of the client's life because the presence of a disability (or, e.g., a sexual-orientation or racial/ethnic difference) leads to the assumption that the issue is unimportant for the client, even though it may be crucial (e.g., sexual activity, relationship concerns, or difficulties presented due to chronic illness). Conversely, the second type of error, an error of commission, occurs when the practitioner assumes, without justification, that an issue should be important for a client because of an identified difference when, in fact, it is not (e.g., self-esteem concerns, illness-related concerns, etc.). Consequently, Kemp and Mallinckrodt suggest that disability-related training in graduate psychology programs should include a minimum of three components: (a) education on the cultural history of people with disabil-ities, including ongoing stereotypes and biases; (b) education on related potential mental health issues (e.g. alienation, discrimination, relation-ship concerns); and (c) training in effective intervention strategies to avoid disruptions in the therapeutic alliance that result from inappropri-ate practitioner behaviors.

Little empirical or theoretical attention has been directed toward de-veloping specific psychotherapeutic interventions for gay men with chronic illness or disability. Exceptions include condition-specific rec-ommendations, such as those for gay men with developmental disabili-ties (Harley, Hall, & Savage, 2000), HIV infection (Treisman & Angelino, 2001), or alcohol dependency (Cheng, 2002). Until empirically derived intervention strategies become available, interventions, theory, and par-adigms created by multicultural counseling and disability scholars need to be examined and modified for use with gay men with chronic illness or disability. Clinicians must remember that such models serve as use-ful heuristics only if the clinician remains curious and does not adopt a "cookie cutter" or "cookbook" approach to treatment. Gay men with disabilities do not comprise a homogeneous group, but are individuals who share common characteristics. It is important to remember that the greatest amount of variance among groups exists within rather than be-tween groups (Aponte, Rivers, & Wohl, 1995). In contrast to stereo-types, which are rigid and usually prevent consideration of difference, generalizations provide a "springboard" for considering the relevance of a particular group attribute or characteristic for an individual within the group. However, generalizations should not be misunderstood as fact.

With this in mind, mental health practitioners should be alert to un-derstanding issues that may confront gay men living with disabil-ity/chronic illness, without compromising the need to avoid stereotypes. Issues that may be particularly salient for gay men with chronic ill-nesses or disability include (a) the impact of illness/disability on sexual functioning, (b) physical overvaluation/idealization, (c) living with a non-life-threatening chronic illness or disability in a community once decimated by HIV, and (d) disclosing sexual identity to potentially ho-mophobic medical providers and patient-support organizations.

Impact of Illness/Disability on Sexual Functioning

Many chronic illness/disabilities may either directly–or through their treatments–affect sexual functioning. For example, medical conditions ranging from spinal cord injury to diabetes can result in erectile dysfunction, while medications for conditions ranging from depression to hypertension may have similar deleterious side effects. As members of a community that tends to place a high value on sexuality, such issues may be particularly troublesome to gay men, both single and partnered.

Physical Overvaluation/Idealization

Effective medical treatments may result in disfiguring changes to one's physical appearance. As is well known, treatment with corticosteroids for autoimmune conditions may result in facial bloating, chemotherapy for cancer may result in hair loss, and treatments for HIV infection can result in facial wasting, accumulation of abdominal fat, or "buffalo hump." Medical providers may perceive the level of disfigurement as negligible; however, gay men may report that such physical changes are more devastating than the illness itself. In a community that tends to emphasize physical attractiveness, any change in appearance can be experienced as profound and may have a significant impact on adherence to treatment.

Living with a Non-Life-Threatening Chronic Illness or Disability in a Community Once Decimated by HIV

As American society ages, more and more people are living with chronic health conditions, such as arthritis, diabetes, glaucoma, or hypertension. Gay men raised in an era when AIDS was almost uniformly fatal have been socialized to regard non-life-threatening, non-HIV-related health concerns as trivial. Gay men may be reluctant to pursue treatment for such conditions, and when the conditions do become the focus of medical attention, feelings of guilt may arise.

Disclosing Sexual Identity to Potentially Homophobic Medical Providers and Patient-Support Organization

Whenever a gay man seeks services from a new medical provider or patient-support organization, he confronts the issue of coming out to the provider/organization. Intake forms inquire about "marital status" and typically offer the heterosexist options of "married" or "single." When listing an emergency contact, the form typically asks the respondent to specify the "relationship." Coming out or withholding information in such situations may add to the already significant stress of seeking treatment or support.

These examples are by no means comprehensive. The intention is to sensitize mental health practitioners to the types of unique concerns and stressors facing gay men with chronic illnesses or disabilities. Practitioners need to remain aware that these and other barriers to obtaining optimal medical care/support may need to be addressed in treatment.

INTERVENTION STRATEGIES AND TECHNIQUES

In a society focused on activities, on doing and fixing, people with chronic illnesses and disabilities are an enigma. We cannot be fixed. We find that generally people want to do something, when what we need is someone just to be near, to accompany us. (Caron, 1996, p. 25)

It is now commonly recognized that effective mental health services for persons with disabilities, and other minority group members, are best achieved when clinicians consider the impact of personal, familial, cultural, societal, and environmental factors (Atkinson & Hackett, 1998; Whyte & Ingstad, 1998). The challenge, of course, is to place the client's day-to-day realities at the center of the therapeutic interaction. Psychoanalysis, cognitive-behavioral, social systems, and other theories of psychology continue to offer important psychotherapeutic strategies (McDowell, Bills, & Eaton, 1991; Thomas & Siller, 1999). However, newer paradigms, which conceptualize sexual orientation and the rehabilitation process within a minority-group and social constructivist perspective (see Garnets, 2002; Livneh, 1991a), remind clinicians to think broadly about disability and suggest the need for an eclectic approach to resolving client concerns. Although no one approach is best for all clients, the biopsychosocial model, which eliminates mind-body dualism, provides a comprehensive understanding of adjustment to chronic illness, disability, and rehabilitation (Feist-Price, 1999).

Hays's (1996a, 1996b) ADRESSING model of assessment reminds clinicians to consider nine significant cultural factors that can impact clients' psychosocial functioning: Age and generational influences; Disability; Religion; Ethnicity; Social status; Sexual orientation; Indigenous heritage; National origin; and Gender. Information gathered through the ADRESSING model allows clinicians to evaluate the contribution of social factors when trying to understand clients' problems in living.

With minor modifications, Paniagua's (1994) recommendations for assessment and intervention with Black clients can be helpful to mental health practitioners working with gay men with disabilities. He suggests that clinicians (a) discuss apparent differences (e.g., disabled vs. nondisabled; straight vs. gay), (b) explore acculturation level (e.g., gay, disability, and racial/ethnic identity development), (c) avoid causal explanations of problems (i.e., recognize the impact of a disabling, homophobic environment), (d) include spirituality and religion in the assessment and therapy process, (e) define the role of those accompanying the client (e.g., family members, significant others, or interpreters), (f) use a present-time focus, (g) screen carefully for depression, (h) avoid misdiagnosing (e.g., by failing to recognize cultural contribution to illness schemas), (i) handle family secrets with care, and provide a safe and trusting environment, and (j) do not try "hard" to understand; rather, be willing to listen and learn from the client.

It is generally accepted that therapeutic success relies on the establishment of a working alliance. Patterson, McKenzie, and Jenkins (1995) recommended that practitioners (a) remember that individuals with disabilities are people, first and foremost, but acknowledge that a disability exists; (b) speak directly to the person with a disability, even when a helper is present; (c) use common words when speaking to individuals with visual impairments or who use wheelchairs ("look," "see," "walk"); and (d) offer assistance to a person with a disability, but wait until it is accepted before providing it. Suggestions for enhancing interactions with people with disabilities are offered by the APA Public Interest Directorate (1999), and include not making assumptions about a person's ability to communicate, speaking at a normal rate and volume, and rephrasing sentences rather than repeating them. Similarly, the President's Committee on Employment of People with Disabilities (1995) offers information on communicating with or writing about people with disabilities. Finally, O'Connor (1993) stressed the need to create partnerships with people with disabilities. The very people who have long been excluded are those best equipped to offer clinicians and researchers insight into how to move forward in partnerships. A practitioner's willingness to listen and provide clients with an opportunity to exercise power, control, and voice will lay the groundwork for an effective therapeutic alliance.

CONCLUSION

Gay men, like all members of society, are at risk for developing chronic illnesses/disabilities. As members of communities already experiencing stress and discrimination, gay men who develop a chronic illness/disability, or people with disabilities who come out as gay may become vulnerable to adjustment problems. Gay men and people with disabilities, unlike members of other minority groups, rarely have family members, neighbors, or important community figures who can validate their experiences, offer advice and support, or serve as role models. Consequently, mental health professionals may be sought out to assist with problems such as identity development, stigma, prejudice, oppression, and discrimination. The interrelationship between the areas of sexual orientation and disability/chronic illness is an area of research that has been greatly under/unexamined, and effective intervention strategies have yet to be validated. Nevertheless, gay men with disability continue to seek out the services of mental health practitioners. Thus, it is incumbent upon providers to provide services that honor and respect a client's worldview. Clinicians employing a social-constructivist approach will have taken a significant step toward developing an ethical approach to providing services to gay men with chronic illnesses or disabilities.

REFERENCES

Adams, M., Bell, L. A., & Griffin, P. (1997). *Teaching for diversity and social justice: A sourcebook*. New York: Routledge.

American Psychological Association Public Interest Directorate (1999). *Enhancing your interactions with people with disabilities* [Brochure]. Washington, DC: Author.

American Psychological Association (2000). Guidelines for psychotherapy with lesbian, gay, and bisexual clients. *American Psychologist, 55*, 1440-1451.

Americans With Disabilities Act of 1990, Pub. L. No. 101-336, § 2, 104 Stat. 328 (1991).

Aponte, J. F., Rivers, R. Y., & Wohl, J. (1995). *Psychological interventions and cultural diversity*. Boston: Allyn and Bacon.

Atkins, D., & Marston, C. (Eds.). (1999). Queer and dis/abled [Special Issue]. *Journal of Gay, Lesbian, and Bisexual Identity, 4*.

Atkinson, D. R., & Hackett, G. (Eds.) (1998). *Counseling diverse populations (2nd ed.)*. Boston: McGraw Hill.

Atkinson, D. R., Morten, G., & Sue, D. W. (Eds.). (1993). *Counseling American minorities: A cross-cultural perspective* (4th ed.). Madison, WI: W.C. Brown & Benchmark.

Atkinson, D. R., Morten, G., & Sue, D. W. (Eds.). (1998). *Counseling American minorities* (5th ed.). Dubuque, IA: McGraw Hill.

Bohan, J. S. (1996). *Psychology and sexual orientation: Coming to terms*. New York: Routledge.

Bohan, J. S., & Russell, G. M. (1999). Conceptual frameworks. In J. S. Bohan & G. M. Russell (Eds.), *Conversations about psychology and sexual orientation* (pp. 11-30). New York: New York University Press.

Campos, P. E., & Goldfried, M. R. (Eds.). (2001). Working with gay, lesbian, and bisexual clients [Special Issue]. *Journal of Clinical Psychology, 57,* 681-693.

Caron, C. (1996). Making meaning out of the experiences of our lives. *Women's Education–Education des femmes, 12* (2), 22-25.

Cheng, Z. (2002). Issues to consider when counseling gay people with alcohol dependency. *Journal of Applied Rehabilitation Counseling, 33,* 10-17.

Corbett, J. (1994). A proud label: Exploring the relationship between disability politics and gay pride. *Disability & Society, 9,* 343-357.

D'Augelli, A. R., & Patterson, C. J. (2001). *Lesbian, gay, and bisexual identities and youth.* New York: Oxford University Press.

Davies, D., & Neal, C. (Eds.). (1996). *Pink therapy: A guide for counselors and therapists working with lesbian, gay, and bisexual clients.* Buckingham, England: Open University Press.

DiPlacido, J. (1998). Minority stress among lesbians, gay men, and bisexuals: A consequence of heterosexism, homophobia, and stigmatization. In G. M. Herek (Ed.), *Stigma and sexual orientation: Understanding prejudice against lesbians, gay men, and bisexuals* (pp. 138-159). Thousand Oaks, CA: Sage.

Fine, M., & Asch, A. (2000). Disability beyond stigma: Social interaction, discrimination, and activism. In K. E. Rosenblum & T. C. Travis (Eds.), *The meaning of difference: American constructions of race, sex and gender, social class, and sexual orientation* (2nd ed., pp. 201-210). New York: McGraw Hill.

Freilich, M., Raybeck, D., & Savishinsky, J. (1991). *Deviance: Anthropological perspectives.* New York: Bergin and Garvey.

Garnets, L. D. (2002). Sexual orientations in perspective. *Cultural Diversity and Ethnic Minority Psychology, 8,* 115-129.

Gill, C. J. (1997). Four types of integration in disability identity development. *Journal of Vocational Rehabilitation, 9,* 39-46.

Gonsiorek, J. C., & Weinrich, J. D. (1991). *Homosexuality: Research implications for public policy.* Newbury Park, CA: Sage.

Gordon, B. O., & Rosenblum, K. E. (2001). Bringing disability into the sociological frame: A comparison of disability with race, sex, and sexual orientation statues. *Disability & Society, 16,* 5-19.

Grant, S. K. (1996). Disability identity development: An exploratory investigation. *Dissertation Abstracts International, 57* (09), 5918B (UMI No. 9704201).

Graves, J. L. (2001). *The Emperor's new clothes: Biological theories of race at the millennium.* New Brunswick, NJ: Rutgers University Press.

Haldeman, D. C. (2001). Psychotherapy with gay and bisexual men. In G. R. Brooks & G. E. Good (Eds.), *The new handbook of psychotherapy and counseling with men: A comprehensive guide to settings, problems, and treatment approaches* (pp. 796-815). San Francisco: Jossey-Bass/Pfeiffer.

Harley, D. A., Hall, M., & Savage, T. A. (2000). Working with gay and lesbian consumers with disabilities: Helping practitioners understand another frontier of diversity. *Journal of Applied Rehabilitation Counseling, 31,* 4-11.

Hays, P. A. (1996a). Culturally responsive assessment with diverse older clients. *Professional Psychology: Research and Practice, 27*, 188-193.

Hays, P. A. (1996b). Addressing the complexities of culture and gender in counseling. *Journal of Counseling and Development, 74*, 332-338.

Henderson, G., & Bryan, W. V. (1997). *Psychosocial aspects of disability* (2nd ed.). Springfield, IL: Charles C. Thomas.

Herdt, G. (1997). *Same sex, different cultures: Exploring gay and lesbian lives.* Boulder, CO: Westview Press.

Kameny, F. E. (1971). Homosexuals as a minority group. In E. Sagarin (Ed.), *The other minorities: Non-ethnic collectivities conceptualized as minority groups* (pp. 50-65). Waltham, MA: Ginn.

Kemp, N. T., & Mallinckrodt, B. (1996). Impact of professional training on case conceptualization of clients with a disability. *Professional Psychology: Research and Practice, 27*, 378-385.

LaPlante, M. P., & Carlson, D. (1996). *Disability in the United States: Prevalence and causes, 1992* (Disability Statistics Report No. 6). Washington, DC: National Institute on Disability and Rehabilitation Research.

Lewis, R. J., Derlega, V. J., Berndt, A., Morris, L. M., & Rose, S. (2001). An empirical analysis of stressors for gay men and lesbians. *Journal of Homosexuality, 42*, 63-88.

Linton, S. (1998). *Claiming disability.* New York: New York University Press.

Linton, S., Mello, S., & O'Neill, J. (1996). Disability studies: Expanding the parameters of diversity (pp. 4-10). *Radical Teacher.* Boston: Boston Women's Teachers' Group.

Livneh, H. (1991a). A unified approach to existing models of adaptation to disability: A model of adaptation. In R. P. Marinelli & A. E. Dell Orto (Eds.), *The psychological and social impact of disability* (3rd ed., pp.111-138). New York: Springer.

Livneh, H. (1991b). On the origins of negative attitudes toward people with disabilities. In R.P. Marinelli & A. E. Dell Orto (Eds.), *The psychological and social impact of disability* (3rd ed., pp. 181-196). New York: Springer.

Longmore, P. K. (September/October 1995). The second phase: From disability rights to disability culture. *The Disability Rag and Resource*, 4-11.

Marinelli, R. P., & Dell Orto, A. E. (Eds.). (1999). *The psychological and social impact of disability* (4th ed.). New York: Springer.

McDowell, W. A., Bills, G. F., & Eaton, M. W. (1991). Extending psychotherapeutic strategies to people with disabilities. In R. P. Marinelli & A. E. Dell Orto (Eds.), *The psychological and social impact of disability* (3rd ed, pp. 249-257). New York: Springer.

O'Connor, S. (1993). *Disability and the multicultural dialogue.* Center on Human Policy, Syracuse University: Author.

O'Keefe, J. (1993). Disability, discrimination, and the Americans With Disabilities Act. *Consulting Psychology Journal, 45*, 3-9.

Olkin, R. (1999). *What psychotherapists should know about disability.* New York: Guilford Press.

O'Neill, T., & Hird, M. J. (2001). Double damnation: Gay disabled men and the negotiation of masculinity. In K. Backett-Milburn & L. McKie (Eds.), *Constructing gendered bodies* (pp. 201-223). London: Palgrave.

Paniagua, F. A. (1994). *Assessing and treating culturally diverse clients: A practical guide*. Thousands Oaks, CA: Sage.

Patterson, J. B., McKenzie, B., & Jenkins, J. (1995). Creating accessible groups for individuals with disabilities. *Journal for Specialists in Group Work, 20*, 76-82.

Perez, R. M., DeBord, K. A., & Bieschke, K. J. (2000). *Handbook of counseling and psychotherapy with lesbian, gay, and bisexual clients*. Washington, DC: American Psychological Association.

Phelps, L. (1998). *Health-related disorders in children and adolescents: A guidebook for understanding and educating*. Washington DC: American Psychological Association.

President's Committee on Employment of People with Disabilities (1995). *Communicating with and about people with disabilities* (Fact Sheet). Washington, DC: Author.

Purnell, L. D., & Paulanka, B. J. (1998). *Transcultural health care: A culturally competent approach*. Philadelphia: F.A. Davis.

Reeve, D. (2000). Oppression within the counseling room. *Disability & Society, 15*, 669-682.

Simon, A. (1998). The relationship between stereotypes of and attitudes toward lesbians and gays. In G. M. Herek (Ed.), *Stigma and sexual orientation: Understanding prejudice against lesbians, gay men, and bisexuals* (pp. 62-81). Thousand Oaks, CA: Sage.

Sue, D. W., Arrendondo, P., & McDavis, R. J. (1992). Multicultural counseling competencies and standards: A call to the profession. *Journal of Counseling and Development, 70*, 477-486.

Thomas, K. R., & Siller, J. (1999). Object loss, mourning, and adjustment to disability. *Psychoanalytic Psychology, 16*, 179-197.

Treisman, G. J., & Angelino, A. F. (2001). Systems review: Mental health. In J. G. Bartlett & J. E. Gallant (Eds.), *Medical management of HIV infection: 2001-2002 edition* (pp. 303-312). Baltimore: Johns Hopkins University.

Vash, C. L. (1981). *The psychology of disability: Springer series on rehabilitation* (Vol. 1). New York: Springer.

Whyte, S. R., & Ingstad, B. (1998). Help for people with disabilities: Do cultural differences matter? *World Health Forum, 19*, 42-46.

World Health Organization (1993). *International classification of impairments, disabilities, and handicaps: A manual of classification relating to the consequences of disease*. Geneva, Switzerland: Author.

The Gay Male Gaze:
Body Image Disturbance
and Gender Oppression Among Gay Men

Mitchell J. Wood

SUMMARY. This article examines body image disturbance among gay men from various sociocultural perspectives. A review of the empirical literature on body image disturbance indicates that gay males experience greater body dissatisfaction than other groups due to their higher levels of gender nonconformity. The impact of gendered power relations on body image is considered in light of feminist, postmodernist, queer, and disability theories of the body. The history of gay bodily beauty is also examined, along with contemporary critiques of gay body politics. The author concludes that gender oppression constitutes a distinct mode of psychosocial oppression among gay men that is no less disabling than heterosexism, and therefore deserves greater attention in gay affirmative theory, research, and practice. *[Article copies available for a fee from The Haworth Document Delivery Service: 1-800-HAWORTH. E-mail address: <docdelivery@haworthpress.com> Website: <http://www.HaworthPress.com> © 2004 by The Haworth Press, Inc. All rights reserved.]*

Mitchell J. Wood, MDiv, MSW, is affiliated with the New York University Ehrenkranz School of Social Work, Columbia University Center for Gay and Lesbian Mental Health.

Address correspondence to: 195 Garfield Place #4E, Brooklyn, NY 11215 (E-mail: mjw245@nyu.edu).

[Haworth co-indexing entry note]: "The Gay Male Gaze: Body Image Disturbance and Gender Oppression Among Gay Men." Wood, Mitchell J. Co-published simultaneously in *Journal of Gay & Lesbian Social Services* (Harrington Park Press, an imprint of The Haworth Press, Inc.) Vol. 17, No. 2, 2004, pp. 43-62; and: *Gay Men Living with Chronic Illnesses and Disabilities: From Crisis to Crossroads* (ed: Benjamin Lipton) Harrington Park Press, an imprint of The Haworth Press, Inc., 2004, pp. 43-62. Single or multiple copies of this article are available for a fee from The Haworth Document Delivery Service [1-800-HAWORTH, 9:00 a.m. - 5:00 p.m. (EST). E-mail address: docdelivery@haworthpress.com].

http://www.haworthpress.com/web/JGLSS
© 2004 by The Haworth Press, Inc. All rights reserved.
Digital Object Identifier: 10.1300/J041v17n02_03

KEYWORDS. Gay men–United States, homosexuality, body image disturbance, body, human–social aspects, power–social sciences, gender identity, feminist theory, postmodern theory, queer theory, disability studies

INTRODUCTION

"Why is it that very time I see a beautiful man I feel self-loathing instead of pleasure?" This is how a gay client in my psychotherapy practice recently articulated his presenting problem. While internalized homophobia might be considered the most obvious explanation for such a complaint, it does not seem to apply in this case, since the client has been out for over two decades, has been a gay rights activist for much of that time, and has made significant cultural contributions that are explicitly gay-positive. Like others in my practice with similar complaints, he reports and evidences a deep acceptance of his homosexuality, while expressing an equally deep dissatisfaction with his experience as a gay man. Although generally these men recognize the profound, pervasive, and pernicious effects of heterosexism, they do not regard it as the primary source of their pain. More often than not, they complain about a chronic sense of inadequacy and isolation they experience within "the gay community." After struggling to accept themselves as gay, and after coming out to family, friends, and work associates, many find themselves in the absurd and agonizing position of now feeling most deeply rejected by other gay men. Because they seem to experience as much alienation and oppression within gay circles as outside of them, heterosexism and homophobia do not adequately address some of the most common complaints and deepest conflicts that uniquely afflict many gay men.

Along with others, the client quoted above expresses much of his self-loathing in terms of feeling physically ugly, sexually undesirable, and invisible among other gay men. He especially hates the shape of his body, believing it will never conform to gay images of beauty, despite spending hours in the gym most days of the week. While condemning the superficial values of those around him, he nonetheless longs to be validated by them, and so habitually measures the worth of himself and others by standards contrary to his own sense of well-being and fairness, making him feel hopelessly trapped in a vicious cycle of unfulfilled desire, envy, and resentment. In my clinical experience, the self-defeating nature and apparent superficiality of these preoccupa-

tions are usually quite evident to those who have them, compounding
the shame and self-blame that already accompanies their intense feelings of inadequacy. They therefore typically regard their problem as
personal in nature, a belief that is prone to reinforcement by significant
others, popular culture, and the individualistic approach of mental
health professionals (Thompson, Heinberg, Altabe, & Tantleff-Dunn,
1999).

This tendency to personalize the problem of poor body image has yet
to be adequately critiqued and challenged by gay men, who have generally failed to pay sustained attention to the social and political dimensions of the problem. Whereas feminists have fought passionately
against the male gaze, many gay men are still fighting passionately for
it, striving to extend its reach, wishing to partake of its power. For those
who feel like chronic losers in the competitive game of the gay male
gaze, there is a dearth of critical discourses within gay communities to
resist its cultural hegemony; and as a result, there is an overabundance
of personal narratives about feeling ugly and inadequate.

Just as sexual minorities have reclaimed their identities and desires
through the ongoing elimination of heterosexism within themselves and
society, the identities of gay men might likewise be strengthened as we
analyze and resist oppressive dynamics among ourselves that foster
widespread patterns of self-loathing. To this end, the remainder of this
article is devoted to the examination of body image disturbance among
gay men from various sociopolitical perspectives. It begins by review-
ing psychological studies on gay men and body dissatisfaction. The focus then turns to various sociocultural theories of the body, after which
historical and contemporary perspectives on gay male body politics are
considered. The concluding section emphasizes the centrality of gendered
power relations to the conceptualization of body image disturbance and
other psychosocial issues relevant to gay men.

BODY IMAGE DISTURBANCE AMONG GAY MEN

Several studies over the last decade have examined body dissatisfaction among gay males, lesbians, straight males, and straight females. Of
all four groups, gay men report the highest levels of body dissatisfaction
(Strong, Singh, & Randall, 2000) or show levels of dissatisfaction com-
parable to straight women and lesbians (Beren, Hayden, Wilfley, &
Grilo, 1996). Other research indicates that lesbians report greater satisfaction than both gay males and straight females, with virtually every

study concurring that straight men are the most satisfied with their bodies (Lakkis, Ricciardelli, & Williams, 1999; Siever, 1996). Compared to heterosexual men, gay males are more likely to binge, purge, and frequently diet (French, Story, Remafedi, Resnick, & Blum, 1996); show greater preoccupation with food and weight (Mishkind, 1986); report more dissatisfaction with body build, waist, biceps, arms, and stomach; have a greater discrepancy between ideal and actual body shapes (Silberstein, Mishkind, Striegel-Moore, Timko, & Rodin, 1989); suffer from low self-esteem and depression (Beren et al., 1996); display higher levels of shame; and exhibit symptomology associated with both subclinical eating pathology and clinical disorders (Beren, 1997). Research also shows that gay teens and bisexual boys are 15 times more likely than heterosexual boys to report binge eating and body image concerns (Gay.com, 2002). Perhaps most discouraging, a study found that affiliation with the gay community is associated with a significant increase in body dissatisfaction (Beren et al., 1996), which does not bode well for teenagers seeking healing and guidance within gay communities.

For the most part, the empirical literature offers two explanations for the greater occurrence of body image disturbance among gay men: objectification and gender nonconformity. The first maintains that gay men and straight women suffer relatively higher levels of body dissatisfaction because both groups desire to be sexually attractive to men. Numerous studies confirm the common belief that men give higher priority to the physical attributes of their romantic partners than women (Siever, 1996). As a result, it is believed that gay men and straight women strive to conform to male images of beauty in order to find partners for sex and romance. Consistent with this hypothesis, research indicates that the experience of objectification by romantic partners is associated with increased emphasis on physical attractiveness, greater body dissatisfaction, more body-related shame, and greater vulnerability to eating disorders (Siever, 1996).

Research has also confirmed the common belief that gay men generally ascribe greater importance to attractiveness than other groups, with physical appearances being more central to their personal and cultural identities. In a study of personal ads placed by men and women (both gay and straight), it was found that men emphasized "objective and physical characteristics," whereas women were more interested in the "psychological aspects of a potential relationship" (Deaux & Hanna, 1984, p. 374). Furthermore, while lesbians placed less emphasis on attractiveness than straight women, gay men distinguished themselves from all other groups by objectifying both themselves and their partners

(Deaux & Hanna, 1984). Research also shows that while men primarily evaluate their bodies in terms of effectiveness, women judge their bodies on the basis of appearances, leading to the hypothesis that the greater incidence of body dissatisfaction among gay men is due to their susceptibility to negative self-assessments in both domains, since they are socialized as men and sexually objectified like women (Siever, 1996). A similar dynamic is seen in studies showing that women want to lose body fat and become thinner, while men want to gain muscle mass and become bigger. Although gay and straight men share the same desire to get bigger, twice as many gay men also want to become thinner, despite the fact they are already slightly lighter on average than straight men. In contrast, lesbians are typically heavier than straight women but are still more satisfied with their bodies (Siever, 1996). Thus, research suggests that the intersection of gender and sexual orientation compounds body dissatisfaction among gay men, since it reinforces their tendency to objectify both themselves and each other, and to judge their bodies by diverging and conflicting standards.

The centrality of gender to body image research is also evident in the explanation of gender nonconformity for body dissatisfaction among gay men. Findings indicate that gay males not only report more body dissatisfaction than other groups but also more childhood gender nonconformity, on account of the high prevalence of "effeminacy" among (pre)homosexual boys (Strong et al., 2000). Research demonstrates that gender nonconformity among males is highly stigmatized, much more so than among females, which may account for the greater frequency of suicide attempts among homosexual boys (Remafedi, 1994). Other studies show that gay men experienced significantly more distress from childhood teasing about physical appearance than all other groups, suggesting causal relationships between childhood gender nonconformity, teasing, and body dissatisfaction (Beren et al., 1996). Most importantly, intergroup differences in body dissatisfaction disappeared when childhood gender nonconformity was statistically controlled (Strong et al., 2000). The primacy of gender over sexual orientation is further supported by data indicating that differences in body dissatisfaction among adult males is much more closely related to gender traits than to sexual orientation (Lakkis et al., 1999). Therefore, body dissatisfaction is perhaps most prevalent among males with female traits, irrespective of their sexual orientation. The tendency within hetero/sexist society to blame these men for symptoms associated with their "effeminate" personalities is mitigated by sociocultural perspectives that identify altogether different sources of their distress.

SOCIOCULTURAL THEORIES OF THE BODY

Body image disturbance is increasingly understood in terms of sociocultural processes (Cash & Pruzinsky, 2002; Thompson et al., 1999). The relevance of social theory to the psychology of body image may be illuminated through the examination of key intellectual movements promoting this recent theoretical shift. Over the last few decades there has been a growing profusion of scholarship in the social sciences and humanities centering on the body (Longhurst, 2001). The first signs of this "somatic turn" in social theory emerged in the 1960s within interdisciplinary studies of health and illness that challenged the biological determinism and reductionism of the medical model, the dominant paradigm of the day. In its place, academics advanced the sociocultural model of health and illness that gives priority to social relations, economic conditions, and cultural norms. This early effort to rescue the body from biomedicine by accentuating its sociocultural context laid the groundwork for the "body craze" that subsequently swept through the academy and beyond (Sabo & Gordon, 1995). Indeed, claims are now made that we live in a "somatic society" in which "major political and personal problems are both problematized within the body and expressed through it" (Turner, 1996, p. 1).

Feminist Bodies

Feminists were the first to produce extensive theory and research that specifically focused on the body as a sociocultural construct (Longhurst, 2001). In the 1970s, the critique of biomedicine was advanced by the women's health movement, as seen in the publication of *Our Bodies, Ourselves* (Boston Women's Health Book Collective, 1971). Feminist scholars resisted the reduction of the body to biological matter, as if it were entirely presocial, ahistorical, and governed by the laws of nature. They instead viewed it as the site of intense sociopolitical struggle. The feminist movement waged legal battles and cultural wars that were specifically body centered, focusing on the right of women to control their bodies in such areas as abortion, rape, domestic violence, and media imagery (Longhurst, 2001). Feminists attacked the naturalization of dichotomous conceptions of sexual differences that subordinated women to men. In doing so, they displaced the notion of biological sex with the idea of gender to signify the social construction of sexuality (Clinchy & Norem, 1998). Along with biomedicine, science itself was subjected to systematic critique and judged to be gender biased. It was argued that scientific research was dominated by men, upheld "man"' as the universal standard from which women deviate, and advanced the male project of objectifying nature for the purpose of domination (Keller, 1985). Many feminists also contended that modern science recapitulated the binary logic–and especially the mind-body dualism–endemic to western civilization, which has associated men with mind, reason, and objectivity, while identifying women with "lower" bodily passions. As a result of this historical legacy, feminists maintain that women have come to experience themselves as objects of the male gaze, leading them to become over-invested in their appearance and to base their self-esteem on conformity to male standards of physical beauty (Cash & Pruzinsky, 2002). In these ways, feminists have primarily attributed women's experiences of body dissatisfaction to gendered power relations evident throughout western philosophical, political, and cultural traditions, rather than ascribing them to individual psychopathology.

Since the late 1980s, feminist gender theories have played an increasingly decisive role in scholarly discourse on men and masculinity (Sabo & Gordon, 1995). In his book on gender and power, Connell (1987) developed the theory of "hegemonic masculinity" to describe the ideology of dominant male groups that not only oppress women but also lesser-status males. He challenges the idea that masculinity is a monolithic entity, such that all men oppress women equally. Instead, he stresses that there are vast differences in the degree to which men may either benefit or suffer from the prevailing gender order, since there are in fact competing masculinities that are hierarchically organized, including hegemonic, marginalized, and stigmatized masculinities. He also views intermale and intersex dominance hierarchies as mutually reinforcing and reflective of one another, as evident in the stigmatization of gay men on account of their identification with women within the existing gender system. Thus, Connell concludes that gender differences not only mediate the domination of men over women but are likewise used by men against men.

Postmodern Bodies

During the 1970s, Foucault instigated the proliferation of poststructuralist discourses on the body and its relation to power (Watson, 2000). While at that time feminists generally conceived of power as massive institutional structures that were both hierarchical and centralized (like the government), Foucault gave priority to the "microphysics" of power, stressing its dispersion throughout the entire body politic and its intimate inscription on the flesh itself (McNay, 1993). Indeed, Foucault (1978) views the body as a product of power dynamics that "reach into the very grain of individuals, touches their bodies and inserts itself into their actions and attitudes, their discourses, learning processes and everyday lives" (p. 39). To explain the origin of these dynamics, Foucault argues that modern science does not discover truth so much as exercise power through the production of knowledge. This power-as-knowledge is then strategically deployed throughout society in the form of scientific discourses, expert techniques, and institutions which discipline and normalize "docile bodies." From a Foucauldian perspective, medical science, clinics, health regimes, gyms, and beauty regimens are all ordinary means by which modern societies subjugate bodies and produce a state of internalized compliance and self-surveillance without the exercise of external control. Despite the ubiquity of these forms of domination, however, Foucault also sees the body as a potential site of localized resistance due to the inherent instability and reversibility of power. In this way, Foucault offers hope for redeployments of power directed toward the construction of new forms of bodily pleasure, diverse modes of human relationship, and alternative technologies of the self (Hancock et al., 2000).

Throughout the 1990s, postmodern scholarship on body politics expanded rapidly, with fluidity and malleability emerging as central metaphors (Longhurst, 2001). The body was no longer a fixed essence, dependent on natural physiological processes, but had become "plastic, a lifestyle accessory, a thing to be sculpted, shaped and stylized," being transformed from a biological fact into a project and performance (Hancock et al., 2000, p. 3). Postmodern theorists note that consumer capitalism tends to reduce depth to surface, identity to image, and ethics to aesthetics, so that "to look good is to feel good is to be good" (Hancock et al., 2000, p. 21). As a result, bodily signs of health and beauty confirm the moral worth of the inner person, while illness and unattractiveness signify a lack of self-control or moral weakness, a semiotic system governed by the underlying principle that beauty is good and ugly is evil. Aesthetic discrimination, therefore, operates as a powerful regulatory force throughout society, serving to stigmatize difference while promoting social conformity and stratification, with some arguing that aesthetic relations are just as determinative of social status as class, gender, race, and ethnicity (Hancock et al., 2000). Indeed, research demonstrates the pervasiveness of appearance stereotypes, as well as the prevalence of stigmatization and discrimination on the basis of these stereotypes. Research also indicates that these prejudicial attitudes and behaviors lead to the internalization of social stigma among persons viewed as unattractive, who predictably exhibit greater signs of distress and psycho-pathology (Cash, 1990). Furthermore, these beauty stereotypes have a strong correlation with gender stereotypes, so that attractive males and females are seen as more masculine and feminine, respectively (Cash, 1990). In postmodern cultures, therefore, gendered body aesthetics are not a superficial or trivial matter, but a fundamental mode of power and domination that have gained the legitimacy and force of an ethical imperative.

Queer Bodies

Along with postmodern feminists, queer theorists explore the fluidity and ambiguity of sex and gender categories, while also giving special attention to the social construction of sexual orientation (Jagose, 1996). With regard to queer conceptions of the body, Kiley (1998) writes:

> The basic idea of most queer body theory is that gay/queer men self-consciously fabricate, then distance themselves from gendered body images. They use tactics of parody and mimicry, thus enabling them through incongruity (butch goes poof) or excess (hypermasculinity and its emblems) to criticize or ironize "normal, standard masculinity." (p. 334)

Many theorists have interpreted camp, drag, and gay machismo as modes of cultural critique and resistance to the prevailing hetero/sexist gender system. They argue that gay men wage "semiotic guerilla warfare" (Weeks, 1985, p. 191) against traditional masculinity through playful exaggeration, theatricalization, and literalization of traditional gender norms (Halperin, 1995). Other theorists, however, seriously doubt the subversive intent and political merits of these practices. Bersani (1988), for one, argues that gay hypermasculinity is based on our tendency to idealize the very representations of masculinity that judge and condemn us, so that gay men's gender practices do not transgress gender norms so much as reinforce and extend them. As a result, he maintains that oppressive gender relations are not only imposed on gay men from without, but also emerge from within in the form of our deepest desires and fantasies; and herein lies our greatest challenge.

Disabled Bodies

Disability studies also help to illuminate the sociocultural dimensions of the body. Over the last few decades, an international movement has politicized disability, transforming it from an individual medical problem into a human rights issue. Similar to black, gay, and women's rights movements, the disability movement is fighting for emancipation from institutionalized oppression, which in this case is called (dis)ablism, a form of discrimination equivalent to racism, sexism, and heterosexism (Oliver, 1996). Along with lesbians and gay men, persons with disabilities have chosen to resist pathologizing discourses and normalizing disciplines, so they too can come out of the closet, take pride in their differences, and demand their rights (Hancock et al., 2000).

Disability theory is grounded in the social model of disability, which above all maintains that society disables individuals, not bodily impairments. The social model is based on a fundamental distinction between impairment and disability, in which impairment denotes physiological disorder in mind or body, while disability refers to restrictions placed on persons with impairments due to social, economic, and political barriers. On the basis of this distinction, the social model maintains that disability is not caused by personal problems and limitations, but is constructed by a disablist society that fails to provide adequate services to meet the basic needs of impaired people, who consequently are marginalized and impoverished. The social model denies any causal relationship between bodily impairment and functional disability, since by definition disability is entirely a function of social (dis)organization. By highlighting the social structural dimensions of disability, the social model defines itself in direct opposition to "the personal tragedy theory" of the medical model, which holds that disability is a random event that happens to unfortunate individuals. The social model instead underscores the fact that disability is not randomly distributed throughout the general population, but is strongly determined by class, race, gender, age, and other material differences (Oliver, 1996).

Since the mid-1990s, however, disabled persons have expressed increasing dissatisfaction with the social model of disability. Those influenced by postmodernism, for instance, have rejected the categorical distinction between impairment and disability, arguing that they are both socially constructed. There is also growing frustration within disability studies and other disciplines with sociocultural theories in general. All are being criticized for promoting a form of social determinism no less rigid and reductionist than biomedical determinism, since they tend to eclipse personal agency and bodily experience (Longhurst, 2001; Watson, 2000). As one author put it, "Contemporary treatment of the body has: mainly been theoretical rather than empirical; focused on the social body rather than the physical body; and tended to interpret the body from an etic (outsider/social science) perspective rather than from an emic (insider/lay) perspective" (Watson, 2000, p. 60). Thus, there is currently an interdisciplinary rebellion against treatment of the body exclusively in terms of structural, metaphorical, or semiotic abstractions.

The quest is now for *embodied* social theory that highlights the interplay between personal agency and social structure. From this perspective, the body is not seen as a unitary entity or text, but as a multidimensional construct: a set of relationships among divergent social discourses and personal experiences (Watson, 2000). While disability studies in the United States emphasizes a holistic, biopsychosocial approach (in which "social" refers to interpersonal, familial, and group levels), British theorists have been more careful to include the societal and structural levels as well (Albrecht, 2002). In this way, theories of embodiment seek to recognize the full weight of social injustice and biomedical conditions, without denying individual and collective powers of resistance and resilience. Similarly, body image disturbance may be seen as derivative of structural oppression, while still affirming our innate capacity for personal transformation.

CONTESTED BODIES AND COMPETING MASCULINITIES AMONG GAY MEN

The History of Gay Beauty

Despite common notions about the self-evident nature of physical beauty, historical and anthropological studies demonstrate that physical attractiveness is a widely variable concept that constantly changes as a direct result of its sociocultural context (Cash & Pruzinsky, 2002). Historians have given much attention to the fluidity of beauty ideals throughout the history of western civilization, especially in relation to women, ranging from the chubby Rubenesque bodies of the sixteenth century to the thin, toned, and busty ideals of today (Thompson et al., 1999). More than biology, research suggests that class is the primary determinant of beauty standards in any given culture, since those with wealth and power are able to obtain that which is most valued within their particular group (Cash & Pruzinsky, 1990).

As with women, a number of historians have traced the development of gay ideals of physical beauty (Chauncey, 1994; D'Emilio, 1983). At the end of the nineteenth century in England and America, the dominant image of beauty among homosexual men was that of the dandy: young, soft, aesthetically sensitive, and effeminate. Prior to the trials of Oscar Wilde, the general public did not particularly associate effeminacy with same-sex acts, so the former was more readily accepted as an alternative style of male appearance and behavior. Thereafter, however, effeminacy became tied to the newly developed concept of the homosexual person, whereby both became heavily stigmatized. As a result, homosexual and heterosexual men alike increasingly masked their feminine traits to avoid association with homosexuality, so the ideal of the dandy fell out of favor. According to Signorile (1997), the denigration of effeminacy persisted throughout the twentieth century, eventually leading to the ascendancy of the hypermasculine iconography of the gay "macho clone" in the 1970s. In the process, the range of acceptable gender styles for sexual object choice were dramatically narrowed throughout gay communities, with the result being that the effeminate homosexual continued to be stigmatized in both gay and straight worlds.

With the advent of the AIDS epidemic in the 1980s, the range of acceptable gender styles narrowed even further, since the "feminine" position in gay sex became identified with death and disease. In response, gay men felt the desperate need to appear healthy and disease-free. To do so, they signaled their identification as "tops" by upholding traditional signs of masculinity, which above all became emblematized in the form of muscle mass. Enormous chests and bulging biceps defended against both actual and symbolic signs of wasting syndrome and disease (Signorile, 1997). Because older gay men became associated with sickness and guilt, the ideal body image became increasingly pubescent and clean-cut, resulting in the idealization of the smooth, hairless body (Signorile, 1997). Regardless of however many subcultural types of masculinity actually existed, the hunky, buff boy came to represent the only gender style openly marketed as a desirable object choice for gay men. To this day, virtually all others–but especially effeminate men–have been rendered as unworthy objects of desire by the monolithic iconography of the gay mass media and cultural industry (Signorile, 1997).

Contemporary Gay Culture Wars

Signorile (1997) argues that even though there are actually many different gay communities, there is nonetheless a body-focused subculture that is increasingly dominating the iconography and institutional culture of gay public life, as seen in gyms, bars, sex clubs, and advertising. He describes this subculture as primarily composed of young, white professionals living in urban ghettoes who above all are bound together by conformity to a very specific ideal: a mesomorphic body type that is "hard, chiseled, buff and smooth" (Mann, 1998, p. 346). Self-identifying watchwords of this subculture include "straight-acting" and "straight-appearing," while "fats," "fems," and "trolls" constitute the demonized Other–unless of course they're serving as the entertainment (Signorile, 1997). Signorile emphasizes that "in postmodern capitalist America, with its hyper-media and ever present advertising bombardment" (p. 31), this commercialized subculture has a powerful impact on most gay men despite its relatively small size, in much the same way that virtually all women are profoundly impacted by the fashion, film, and beauty industries. Along with others, Signorile calls this gay caste system a form of "body oppression" or "body fascism," which he defines as "a rigid set of standards of physical beauty that pressures everyone within a particular group to conform to them" (p. 27-28). As he puts it:

> In a culture in which the physical body is held in such high esteem and given such power, body fascism then not only deems those who don't or can't conform to be sexually less desirable, but in the extreme–sometimes dubbed "looksism"–also deems an individual completely worthless *as a person*, based solely on his exterior. In this sense it is not unlike racism or sexism or homophobia itself. (p. 28)

Signorile goes on to describe how this subculture is based on a "cult of masculinity," which finds its purest expression in circuit parties that regularly take place across the country and around the world. It is here that Signorile sees the convergence of the worst features of gay social life: the most rigid and exclusionary physical images of masculinity; the widespread use and abuse of testosterone, anabolic steroids, and human growth hormones to actualize these images; and the nearly universal use and abuse of drugs, especially Ecstasy ("X"), ketamine ("Special K"), GHB ("G"), amphetamines ("crystal meth" or "speed"), and cocaine. He makes reference to research demonstrating the high correlation among steroid use; alcohol and substance use; aggressive and destructive behaviors; eating disorders; excessive workouts; and muscle dysmorphia, a subtype of body dysmorphic disorder characterized by a pathological preoccupation with muscularity. Signorile also notes other important influences on gay images of beauty, including the gay porn industry and various technological advances, including better gym equipment, new drugs and food supplements for muscle growth, and innovative forms of cosmetic surgery for men. Due to these developments, he concludes that the fascistic notion of "genetic superiority" is no longer sufficient to attain the gay ideal of beauty, since

> the ideal was no longer something that occurred in nature. It was a completely manufactured man, an artificially created version of masculinity. The masculine body type that was now most revered could perhaps only be attained by surgery, drug use, and computer enhancement of images. (p. 69)

Rofes (1998) rejects Signorile's characterization of "circuit boys" and the "cult of masculinity." He instead maintains that Signorile stereotypes and scapegoats circuit boys, whipping up the same sort of moral panic that has been used against sexual outsiders for decades now, especially during times of social upheaval. Rofes also criticizes the tendency to place one subculture central stage, as if it represented all gay men, rather than emphasizing the diversity of subcultures, including "bears, men of color, AIDS activists, club kids, trannies, queers, leathermen, or youth" (p. 143), each with its own images of masculinity. As for the cult of masculinity, Rofes contends that Signorile "mistakes culture for cult" (p. 190) and therefore does not show due respect for cultural differences. In fact, rather than decry the supposed body fascism of the cult of masculinity, Rofes believes gay men who fit "traditional masculine conventions" are more likely to suffer discrimination, since "a profound distrust of conventional masculinities pervades [gay] community life" (p. 190-191). Above all, however, Rofes resists the simplification and externalization of social problems that contribute to scapegoating, not only because the demonization of others is intrinsically wrong, but also because it precludes the identification and remediation of the real, underlying problems, which always entail more complexity and complicity than we care to admit. In short, Rofes refuses to participate in "the game of 'good gay/bad gay' that has plagued queers for a very long time," stating flatly that "nothing good comes of it" (p. 144).

This debate between Rofes and Signorile suggests the following question: How can we continue to build respect for our personal and subcultural differences without turning a blind eye to the reality of oppressive and disabling dynamics among gay men? While not attempting to provide a conclusive answer, I nonetheless argue in the final section that any satisfactory response must give central attention to gender oppression, which serves as a deep source of both conflict and commonality among gay men.

CONCLUSION: GENDER OPPRESSION AMONG GAY MEN

Body image disturbance has become a form of normative discontent among gay men who, along with women, can trace the roots of their body dissatisfaction and its disabling effects to gendered power relations instigated and maintained by men. As a result, the body itself has become a crucial site of social struggle, not only between men and women but also between dominant masculinities and subordinate male gender styles that are marginalized and stigmatized. While these oppressive dynamics are clearly based on hetero/sexist ideologies that stigmatize women, homosexuality, and gender nonconformity, they nonetheless have assumed a life of their own within gay social circles, where gender oppression is not merely reenacted but actively reconstructed, revitalized, and redeployed throughout gay cultural life. Just as it is an illusion to imagine that "the gay community" constitutes an organic unity, it is also naïve to believe that "gay communities" are simply composed of benign cultural differences. Rather, gay subcultures occupy positions of power in relation to each other, with some being dominant and others subordinate within the greater context of gay public life. Thus, along with race, class, ethnicity, age, and disability, gendered body aesthetics not only constitute a pivotal dimension in the construction of gay subcultural identities, but also determine power relations both within and between gay subcommunities.

Unlike feminist and lesbian cultures, however, gay men lack a strong tradition of critical analysis of power relations within their communities to complement systematic critiques of heterosexism. This lack of self-critical analysis has persisted because many gay men are still deeply identified with the gendered hierarchies endemic to patriarchal culture. On the one hand, many gay men derive their sense of power from the stigmatization of female traits, while many others are still too constrained by self-stigmatization and shame to confront their own gender oppression. Furthermore, gay men have yet to develop adequate language and theory by which to describe and analyze oppressive gender dynamics among themselves. To date, gay studies have primarily relied on heterosexism and homophobia to conceptualize the psychosocial and political context of gay men (Ritter & Terndrup, 2002). While both concepts are necessary to the theorization of gay lives, they are not sufficient. By definition, heterosexism and homophobia make sexual orientation instead of gender the central category of analysis (Herek, 1996), and, therefore, they do not give primary attention to the core issue of gender oppression that pervades the lives of virtually all gay men.

To achieve greater balance, lesbian theorists widely utilize the concepts of sexism, gynophobia, and misogyny alongside sexual orientation to give equal attention to gender dynamics (D'Augelli & Patterson, 1994). Insofar as these concepts refer to sex role stereotypes and female traits (as opposed to females themselves), they might properly be used to specify gender oppression among gay men. Nonetheless, gay theorists have not made extensive use of them because the terms are primarily associated with the oppression of women by men. While heterosexism, homophobia, sexism, gynophobia, and misogyny are all related to gender oppression among gay men, none of them give primary place to the central issue of stigmatization and discrimination based on gender, without implicit subordination to the categories of biological sex or sexual orientation. Given that gender oppression has a *primary* impact on nearly all gay men, this leaves a significant gap in our capacity to understand and theorize our lives, hindering our ability to accurately identify and overcome the sources of our oppression.

More fundamental than the problem of theory, however, is that of language. We have yet to develop adequate terminology by which to articulate gay male gender identities, since our discourse continues to be rooted in assumptions that are categorically hetero/sexist. This makes it almost impossible to discuss gay men's gender issues without slipping into derogatory, confused, or vague terminology. For example, "effeminacy" is by definition a pejorative term, and so it is best avoided altogether. "Femininity" is also frequently avoided because of its essentialist connotations. "Female traits" is completely inaccurate with reference to men, since the whole point is that these traits are no less male than female. The notion of alternative masculinities is problematic as well, since the concept of "masculinity" (like "manly" or even "man" itself) is deeply implicated in hetero/sexist ideologies. "Gender nonconformity" represents a useful strategic maneuver that manages to avoid all of the above problems, although it does so at the expense of being reduced to a negative concept that lacks specificity. As a result, it is no surprise that gay men resist open discussion and sustained exploration of gender identity issues, since language itself presses us to engage in self-stigmatization, thereby reinforcing feelings of shame rather than helping to release them.

Gay men have avoided dealing with gender oppression, not because it is less important than heterosexism or homophobia, but because it is the deeper issue, more closely associated with personal trauma. In human development, gender identity emerges well before sexual orientation, with gay males generally following a line of gender development from childhood into adulthood that is very different from straight males (Laird & Green, 1996). Due to our gender nonconformity, we generally experience stigmatization based on gender long before discrimination based on sexual orientation (Rottnek, 1999). In this way, sexism lies at the root of heterosexism and gynophobia at the heart of homophobia, so that gender oppression is frequently a source of our deepest wounds. As one of my clients put it, "Nobody cares that I'm a homosexual anymore. What they really can't stand is that I'm effeminate." Even though this client initiated an antidiscrimination lawsuit that eventually set a national precedent for gay rights–demonstrating his first-hand awareness of heterosexism and its devastating effects–he nonetheless believes he has been most deeply damaged by the stigmatization of his "effeminacy." Most sadly, however, he too suspects he is "defective," with his primal flaw being gender nonconformity, not sexual orientation. Most clinicians would probably agree that gender issues are much more pervasive and profound than those of sexual orientation among gay men, with internalized gender oppression being more debilitating than internalized homophobia. Nonetheless, gay affirmative clinical literature ordinarily treats gender trauma and gender oppression as secondary to heterosexism, when in most cases it is actually the other way around. This tendency to minimize gender and subsume it within sexual orientation is not only a byproduct of gay men's deep engagement in the political struggle against heterosexism, but also a product of our tendency to suppress and deny the painful reality of gender trauma and gender oppression within our own lives and communities.

Gender will continue to be a fundamental and irreducible mode of oppression among gay males so long as parents continue to be ashamed of their queer children; "sissies" are subjected to harassment at school without adult intervention or protection; gay teens are pushed to suicide in grossly disproportionate numbers; gay men feel ashamed of their bodies; anal receptivity remains stigmatized even among gay men; hypermasculinity dominates gay mass media and gay public life; and gay men prefer to be "straight-acting" rather than being themselves. As it is now, research associates higher gender nonconformity with character disorders among boys, and in such a way that unduly pathologizes children rather than addressing toxic environments (Rottnek, 1999). We are just beginning to understand the extent to which gender oppression afflicts gay men. Clearly, more empirical research is needed to help elucidate these issues.

In spite of all these challenges, however, language, theory, and culture are currently in the process of being transformed to better account for our gendered experiences. The cultural zeitgeist is moving beyond issues of women and sexism, beyond homosexuality and heterosexism, to now include transgendered persons and gender discrimination as well. Since the negative effects of gender oppression is immediately relevant to women, bisexuals, homosexuals, and transgendered persons alike, our increasing awareness of gender dynamics allows us to further link our diverse identities and divergent politics, further illuminating the interdependence of our struggles for justice.

REFERENCES

Albrecht, G. (2002). American pragmatism, sociology and the development of disability studies. In C. Barnes, M. Oliver, & L. Barton (Eds.), *Disability studies today.* Malden, MA: Blackwell Publishers Inc.

Beren, S. E. (1997). Stigmatization and shame as determinants of subclinical eating disorder pathology: A comparison of gay and heterosexual men. *Dissertation Abstracts International, 58*(4-B), 2109.

Beren, S. E., Hayden, H. A., Wilfley, D. E., & Grilo, C. M. (1996). The influence of sexual orientation on body dissatisfaction in adult men and women. *International Journal of Eating Disorders, 20,* 135-141.

Bersani, L. (1988). Is the rectum a grave? In D. Crimp (Ed.), *AIDS: Cultural analysis, cultural activism.* Cambridge: MIT Press.

Boston Women's Health Book Collective, The (1971). *Our bodies, ourselves.* New York: Simon and Schuster.

Cash, T. & Pruzinsky, T. (Eds.). (1990). *Body images: Development, deviance, and change.* New York: The Guilford Press.

Cash, T. & Pruzinsky, T. (Eds.). (2002). *Body image: A handbook of theory, research, and clinical practice.* New York: The Guilford Press.

Chauncey, G. (1994). *Gay New York: Gender, urban culture, and the making of the gay male world, 1890-1940.* New York: BasicBooks.

Clinchy, B. M. & J. K. Norem, (Eds.). (1998). *The gender and psychology reader.* New York: New York University Press.

Connell, R. W. (1987). *Gender and power: Society, the person, and sexual politics.* Stanford, CA: Stanford University Press.

D'Augelli, A. & Patterson, C. (Eds.). (1994). *Lesbian, gay and bisexual identities over the lifespan: Psychological perspectives.* New York: Oxford University Press.

D'Emilio, J. (1983). Sexual politics, sexual communities: The making of a homosexual minority in the United States, 1940-1970. Chicago: University of Chicago Press.

Deaux, K. & Hanna, R. (1984). Courtship in the personals column: The influence of gender and sexual orientation. *Sex Roles: A Journal of Research, 11*(5-6), 363-375.

Foucault, M. (1978). *The history of sexuality, vol. I: An introduction.* Harmondsworth: Penguin.

French, S. A., Story, M., Remafedi, G., Resnick, M. D., & Blum, R. W. (1996). Sexual orientation and prevalence of body dissatisfaction and eating disordered behaviors:

A population-based study of adolescents. *International Journal of Eating disorders, 19*, 119-126.

Gay.com/Planetout.com Network (2002, October 14). *Being gay affects teens' body image.* Retrieved October 20, 2003, from http://gay.com/news/article.html?2002/10/14/1

Halpern, D. M. (1995). *Saint Foucault: Towards a gay hagiography.* New York: Oxford University Press.

Hancock, P., Hughes, B., Jagger, E., Paterson, K., Russell, R., Tulle-Winton, E., & Tyler, M. (2000). *The body, culture and society: An introduction.* Philadelphia: Open University Press.

Herek, G. (1996). Heterosexism and homophobia. In R. P. Cabaj & T. S. Stein (Eds.), *Textbook of homosexuality and mental health* (pp. 101-114). Washington D.C.: American Psychiatric Press.

Jagose, A. (1996). *Queer theory: An introduction.* New York: New York University Press.

Keller, E. (1985). *Reflections on gender and science.* New Haven, CT: Yale University Press.

Kiley, Dean (1998). Queer crash test dummies: Theory, ageing, and embodied problematics. In D. Atkins (Ed.), *Looking Queer: Body image and identity in lesbian, bisexual, gay and transgender communities* (pp. 327-244). New York: The Haworth Press, Inc.

Laird, J. & Green, R. J. (Eds.). (1996). *Lesbians and gays in couples and families: A handbook for therapists.* San Francisco: Jossey-Bass.

Lakkis, J., Ricciardelli, L. A., & Williams, R. J. (1999). Role of sexual orientation and gender-related traits in disordered eating. *Sex Roles, 41*(1-2), 1-16.

Longhurst, Robyn (2001). *Bodies: Exploring fluid boundaries.* New York: Routledge.

Mann, W. J. (1998). Laws of desire: Has our imagery become over idealized? In D. Atkins (Ed.), *Looking queer: Body image and identity in lesbian, bisexual, gay and transgender communities.* New York: The Haworth Press, Inc.

McNay, L. (1993). *Foucault & feminism: Power, gender and the self.* Boston: Northeastern University Press.

Oliver, M. (1996). *Understanding disability: From theory to practice.* New York: St. Martin's Press.

Ritter, K. Y. & Terndrup, A. I. (2002). *Handbook of affirmative psychotherapy with lesbians and gay men.* New York: The Guilford Press.

Rofes, E. E. (1998). *Dry bones breathe: Gay men creating post-AIDS identities and cultures.* New York: The Haworth Press, Inc.

Rottnek, M. (1999). *Sissies and tomboys: Gender nonconformity and homosexual childhood.* New York: New York University Press.

Sabo, D. & Gordon, D. F. (Eds.). (1995). *Men's health and illness: Gender, power, and the body.* Thousand Oaks: Sage Publications.

Siever, M. D. (1996). The perils of sexual objectification: Sexual orientation, gender, and socioculturally acquired vulnerability to body dissatisfaction and eating disorders. In C. J. Alexander (Ed.), *Gay and lesbian mental health: A sourcebook for practitioners* (pp. 201-226). New York: The Haworth Press, Inc.

Signorile, M. (1997). *Life outside: The Signorile report on gay men: Sex, drugs, muscles, and the passages of life.* New York: Harper Collins Publishers.

Silberstein, L. R., Mishkind, M. E., Striegel-Moore, R. H., Timko, C., & Rodin, J. (1989). Men and their bodies: A comparison of homosexual and heterosexual men. *Psychosomatic Medicine, 51,* 337-346.

Strong, S. M., Singh, D., Randall, P. K. (2000). Childhood gender nonconformity and body dissatisfaction in gay and heterosexual men. *Sex Roles: A Journal of Research, 43*(7-8), 427-439.

Thompson, J. D., Heinberg, L. J., Altabe, M., & Tantleff-Dunn, S. (1999). *Exacting beauty: Theory, assessment, and treatment of body image disturbance.* Washington, DC: American Psychological Association.

Turner, B. S. (1996). *The body and society: Explorations in social theory.* London: Sage.

Watson, J. (2000). *Male bodies: Health, culture, and identity.* Philadelphia: Open University Press.

Weeks, J. (1985). *Sexuality and its discontents: Meanings, myths and modern sexualities.* Boston: Routledge.

The Multidimensional Challenge of Psychotherapy with HIV Positive Gay Men

Ronald J. Frederick

SUMMARY. In the early 1980s, the presenting issues of HIV positive gay men in psychotherapy most often centered on loss, death and dying, but with the advent of protease inhibitors, these clients often present with a different set of issues related to living longer and healthier lives with HIV. In this chapter, the author, a psychologist who has worked with gay men for over a decade, will identify and discuss both the current issues faced by HIV positive gay men as well as the clinical challenges facing therapists who work with this population. Implications for working with gay men with other chronic conditions are considered. *[Article copies available for a fee from The Haworth Document Delivery Service: 1-800-HAWORTH. E-mail address: <docdelivery@haworthpress.com> Website: <http://www.HaworthPress.com> © 2004 by The Haworth Press, Inc. All rights reserved.]*

KEYWORDS. AIDS, clinical practice, health, HIV, HIV positive, mental health, psychosocial issues, psychotherapy

---

Ronald J. Frederick, PhD, LP, is affiliated with the Abbott Northwestern Hospital, Adult Day Health Center.

Address correspondence to: 3100 West Lake Street, Suite 107, Minneapolis, MN 55416 (E-mail: beyerfred@mn.rr.com).

[Haworth co-indexing entry note]: "The Multidimensional Challenge of Psychotherapy with HIV Positive Gay Men." Frederick, Ronald J. Co-published simultaneously in *Journal of Gay & Lesbian Social Services* (Harrington Park Press, an imprint of The Haworth Press, Inc.) Vol. 17, No. 2, 2004, pp. 63-79; and: *Gay Men Living with Chronic Illnesses and Disabilities: From Crisis to Crossroads* (ed: Benjamin Lipton) Harrington Park Press, an imprint of The Haworth Press, Inc., 2004, pp. 63-79. Single or multiple copies of this article are available for a fee from The Haworth Document Delivery Service [1-800-HAWORTH, 9:00 a.m. - 5:00 p.m. (EST). E-mail address: docdelivery@haworthpress.com].

http://www.haworthpress.com/web/JGLSS
© 2004 by The Haworth Press, Inc. All rights reserved.
Digital Object Identifier: 10.1300/J041v17n02_04

Since the early 1980s, psychotherapists working with gay men have been challenged to respond to the ever-changing needs of people living with HIV/AIDS. In the early years of the epidemic, presenting issues most often centered on loss, death and dying. Then, in the mid-1990s, with the advent of protease inhibitors, clients began to present with a different set of issues centered mainly on the fundamental question, "Who am I and what am I going to do with my life now that death may not be imminent?" Now, more than two decades into the HIV/AIDS epidemic, as HIV seems to be transforming from a terminal to a chronic illness, the clinical issues with which clients are presenting in psychotherapy continue to evolve and change. In this chapter, the author, a psychologist who has worked with gay men for over a decade, will identify and discuss both the current issues faced by HIV positive gay men as well as the clinical challenges facing therapists who work with this population in the context of the shifting status of HIV from a decidedly terminal to a chronic illness.

OVERVIEW OF CHANGES IN CLINICAL ISSUES

The first decade of the AIDS crisis was characterized by an atmosphere of despair. A diagnosis of HIV/AIDS was viewed as a death sentence, as few options for treatment were known or available. For mental health practitioners, clinical work with clients with HIV/AIDS largely centered on grief and loss (Gabriel, 1996; Green & Sherr, 1989). Clients came to therapy struggling to come to terms with their lives being dramatically cut short, their bodies being quickly ravaged in ways they had never imagined, and an overwhelming sense of grief as entire networks of family and friends were decimated. Clinicians were forced to stare death in the face as well, to grapple with a multitude of losses, and to struggle with their own mortality and sense of vulnerability. Hope was a commodity hard to come by, and many dared not risk having it.

Then, in the mid-1990s, protease inhibitors burst on the scene. This new class of antiretroviral medication, served up in a "cocktail" that included two different additional HIV meds (nucleoside analogues), miraculously lowered the viral load of HIV in the bloodstream, seemed to restore health, and showed the promise of prolonging life in people with HIV. Clinical issues encountered in therapy shifted away from facing one's demise to facing the prospect of life (Brashers et al., 1999; Farber & McDaniel, 1999). While many gay men were thrilled to be feeling better and able to do things they had longed to do, others presented with ambivalence about a whole new set of conflicts. As one client poignantly explained, "I've spent so long preparing for my death; it's not so easy to start thinking about the possibility of life. And besides, what do I have to live for? Practically all my friends are dead and my family has pulled away, my credit cards are maxed out and I'm totally in debt."

For some gay men who had experienced identity conflict before AIDS, they found in this disease a hook on which to hang a new, more clearly defined self. The result was an interesting paradox–while many men made some positive personal changes as a result of their illness, an identity forged in the absence of something, or in something being taken away, can be problematic. For instance, one patient made dramatic changes in his life after being diagnosed HIV positive. He became sober after years of substance abuse and took steps to address his health, putting himself on a regimen that included exercise, a new diet and getting plenty of rest. He began volunteering for an AIDS organization, joined a PWA support group, and made friends with people who shared his experience. From his point of view, protease inhibitors or, more specifically, a life "without" the immanent death threat of HIV, threatened to take away a sense of meaning in his life–his reason for living. "Who am I now that death has taken a holiday?"

As clinicians, we struggled with whether to accept the "good news" as real or hype. As my clients struggled to make sense of the plethora of emotional and psychological issues that emerged during this time, I found myself also struggling as their therapist. When patients seemed less threatened by HIV, there was a part of me that wanted to join them in their thinking. When patients resisted going on medications, I sometimes became frustrated. And when patients became hopeful, I sometimes felt the impulse to rein them in. In light of much uncertainty, I was filled with questions and doubt–Could this change really last? Would the new meds bring sustainable change? Are there side effects? Is this the end of AIDS?

As time progressed, it became clear that the life expectancy of some people living with HIV/AIDS (that is–those who are able to receive, afford and benefit from up-to-date medical care) could be lengthened through drug treatment that slows the damage HIV does to the immune system. Recent years have brought forth a number of other "new and improved" drug regimens that have answered the prayers of some, but have not offered the same stellar results to others. In addition, currently more than half of HIV-positive people in the United States who are undergoing treatment are infected with strains of the virus that are resistant to one or more antiretroviral drugs (Stephenson, 2002). Of those who have been fortunate enough to experience the sustained benefits of current drug therapies, many have also become plagued by an array of adverse complications and side effects. While there is still much that remains to be understood about the impact of new drug therapies and much room for improvement, at the moment, HIV appears to be shifting toward being a chronic rather than a terminal illness.

As a result, the issues that gay men with HIV/AIDS are now presenting with in psychotherapy run the gamut from those encountered at the beginning of the epidemic when the disease was relatively acute, to those encountered by people living with many other chronic, debilitating, and life-threatening illnesses. More specifically, while issues of complicated grief, loss, and mortality still exist, others such as dealing with varied complications and medication related side effects, medication adherence, sexual negotiations, cognitive deterioration, a change in social status for gay men from "special" to "ordinary," and exhaustion and apathy, can feel, and often are, more immediately paramount. Moreover, as the disease has become more chronic in nature, other nonmedical issues may begin to emerge in treatment that were heretofore masked by a focus on HIV/AIDS. In these cases, the impact of being HIV positive is often overshadowed by other, more long-standing psychosocial issues (Weiss, 1997). Consequently, therapists working with HIV positive gay men are now faced with a more complicated differential diagnosis and an even wider scope of treatment concerns. It is this range of issues to which I now turn my attention.

CURRENT CLINICAL ISSUES

HIV Drug-Related Side Effects

As mentioned earlier, HIV/AIDS medical treatment is not without drawbacks. While medications can be very effective in lowering viral load, they can also bring with them insidious side effects. These complications include but are not limited to fatigue; depression; anemia; digestive problems; diarrhea; HIV-Associated Lipodystrophy Syndrome (abnormal fat distribution from arms, legs and face to stomach and behind the neck; cholesterol and glucose abnormalities which may increase the risk of heart attack or stroke); mitochondrial toxicity (damage to cells which can cause neuropathy or kidney damage, as well as a buildup of lactic acid in the body); bone problems; and liver failure (NIAID, 2002).

As with all chronic diseases, such side effects give rise to a multitude of psychosocial issues (Farber & McDaniel, 1999). Clients struggle with feelings about drug treatment: whether to starts meds, when to start, and whether to stay on meds that are making them feel miserable. Furthermore, side effects loom large in the negotiation of simple daily life. For instance: How do I integrate chronic bouts of diarrhea into my life? How far can I safely be away from a restroom before I have an accident? Can I go back to work when I'm always so tired? Can I actually make plans and stick to them? On an intimate note: How do I feel about my body image? Negotiating intimacy? Going on a date? Having a relationship with someone? In the sexual arena: How do I negotiate safer sex? Do I always need to use condoms? What if I have an undetectable viral load or if my partner is also HIV positive?

In order to be able to understand the choices and experiences with which a client is presented, and to be able to make a differential diagnosis when trying to understand presenting symptoms, therapists working with HIV positive gay men must have a comprehensive understanding of HIV disease and its prevention, as well as an up-to-date working understanding of the effects of drug treatment. Additionally, turning to the literature on other chronic illnesses may provide useful information and transferable guidelines for addressing adjustment to illness. For example, therapists can help clients sort through the issues that arise around deciding whether to start treatment. As a client considers starting meds, or while taking meds begins to experience possible bodily changes, straightforward discussion of body image, processes, functioning and responses should be initiated as an integral part of treatment (Goodheart & Lansing, 1997). In addition, to make matters more complicated, current medical perspectives on the timing and duration of drug treatment differ. Some experts have begun to wonder when it is safe to take patients off of HIV drugs in an effort to lessen complication rates (Zuger, 2002).

Therapists will need to facilitate a respectful, informed, exploration of what can be a very difficult decision-making process as well as be comfortable managing the ambiguity and uncertainty surrounding the disease and treatment. Moreover, drug complications and related symptoms, while physically debilitating, also have a profound effect on one's emotional and psychological well-being. Clients may need assistance as they navigate and address questions about their quality of life and whether to continue treatment. Should a client decide to continue drug treatment, therapeutic work will need to focus on finding a way to adapt to these changes, a process that almost always necessitates grieving over lost functioning as well as changes in physical appearance (Tiamson, 2002).

Fear of Cognitive Deterioration

Because HIV is able to enter the central nervous system early in the course of infection, cognitive impairment is a possible issue for HIV positive gay men (Budin, 1997). Many HIV positive gay men report that their greatest fear in living with HIV is "losing my mind." One member of an HIV support group I facilitate stated that he could handle most of what could happen to him due to HIV, but if he were to become severely impaired cognitively, he would rather end his life. This is a viewpoint shared by most of the other group members. Clinicians working with HIV positive gay men should encourage clients to put words to these HIV-related fears as too often they go unspoken and, as a result, become more intense. Therapists can encourage clients to face their fears by imagining what their experience would be like should they develop dementia. In response, therapists can provide information to help clients more accurately understand the disease process and the kind of changes associated with dementia. This information can go a long way in decreasing one's fears and concerns (Buckingham & Van Gorp,1999). Preemptively identifying and developing strategies to cope with cognitive impairments can help the client feel more in control. In addition, clinicians may need to examine their own possible issues of fear and denial that could impede or prevent these essential discussions. Finally, borrowing from the expertise and information that has been developed with regard to the role of dementia in other disease processes can offer useful insight for both patient and therapist alike in negotiating concerns related to cognitive impairment.

Stigmatization

While all chronic illnesses, to varying degrees, bring with them the burden of stigma, HIV has been unique in this regard due, in large part, to the modes of transmission (mainly through sexual contact and IV drug use). For a while, outward physical signs of HIV/AIDS had all but disappeared and HIV positive gay men could "pass" unidentified. In addition, some gay men enjoyed the physical enhancement that steroids, ostensibly used to combat wasting, gave to their physique, offering them a chance to live out a fantasy of a physical ideal lauded by a influential faction of the gay community. This honeymoon was short-lived. As previously noted, one of the distressing side effects of HIV drugs includes *lipodystrophy*–visible changes in body shape and appearance due to fat redistribution. Outward signs of lipodystrophy include sunken cheeks in the face, increased fat in the face, prominent veins in the legs, loss of fat in the legs and arms, loss of shape in the buttocks, increased fat around the gut, breast enlargement, and/or a fat pad on the back of the neck (sometimes called a *buffalo hump*). Although some aspects of this phenomenon were seen in the earlier years of the epidemic, they are now occurring with more prominence. The "face" of HIV/AIDS has returned in full force, and while cosmetic procedures are being developed and utilized to ameliorate visual changes (by those who can afford them), the internal effects are still present.

For the HIV positive gay man, these physical changes give rise to a multitude of psychosocial stressors among which stigma factors prominently. Given some of the untoward effects of drug treatment, it is not surprising that many gay men living with HIV/AIDS grapple with questions about whether to start or to continue treatment. As one client states, "I see how those people look [with lipodystrophy] . . . like zombies . . . so, I'm supposed to be happy that I can take medication, feel miserable and watch my body fall apart?" In addition to the emotional/psychological toll of a physical assault to their bodies, clients report worrying about how they are perceived by others, and fears of being labeled, shunned, discriminated against, and blamed. Their sense of self may be shaken and social confidence diminished. As one of my clients poignantly explained, "I feel like a leper . . . like I'm defective, damaged goods or something . . . like people look at me and think 'he has AIDS, how did that happen, I mean in this day and age?'" This viewpoint speaks not only to a sense of being stigmatized, but also to another issue faced by those who have been more recently infected. Some gay men experience feelings of culpability for contracting HIV at a time when so much is known about prevention. Consider the case of Tom:

> Tom, a gay man in his early 50s, sought individual psychotherapy to cope with overwhelming anxiety. He was diagnosed HIV positive only months before seeking treatment after years of "playing safe." Tom was full of shame and guilt for becoming infected, unable to acknowledge the antecedents to his putting himself at risk. Long-standing intrapsychic conflict involving his family of origin (unresolved anger and rage toward his emotionally and physically abusive mother and passive, absent father) had to be addressed first, before we were able to make any ground in his developing a more realistic perception of himself and of his being HIV positive. As Tom's perception of himself began to change, he came to see

how depressed and distraught he had been and how his prior self-destructive behavior was unconsciously motivated. He could acknowledge and feel good about the many years he had been able to protect himself from infection. He felt remorse for what he had done, but also compassion for himself, a man who had at one time been so conflicted and who did not "deserve" a horrible illness because of a lapse in judgment.

As therapists working with HIV-positive gay men we need to be aware of and reflect on our ideas and beliefs about HIV/AIDS, as well as the thoughts and feelings engendered in us when directly faced with visual manifestations of HIV infection. It is not uncommon for any of us to have prejudicial perceptions toward conditions that are threatening and give rise to our own personal anxieties and sense of vulnerability (Goodheart & Lansing, 1997). These feelings are heightened when signs of the disease become more evident. For instance, do we hold the patient responsible for being infected? Is a facet of this view accurate? We may need to examine our own preconceptions and biases when necessary so that we can effectively help clients disentangle what may be a healthy sense of remorse around contracting HIV from separate, deep-seated psychological distress which, often times, preceded seroconversion.

Change in Social Status

An issue particular to living with HIV, as opposed to other chronic illnesses, is what might be understood as a change in social status. While the initial public response to AIDS may have been slow, the activism and efforts of many during the early years brought about an explosion of media attention and public response. People took to the streets to fight for needed research, monies and drug approval. For a while AIDS achieved a certain cachet in the media as celebrities donned red ribbons and spoke out for the cause. A staggering array of programs was developed across the country to address a plethora of needs and issues. People living with HIV received free services from AIDS service organizations including but not limited to counseling and social work services, home visits and practical support, legal assistance, nutritional counseling, workshops, classes, social events, complimentary therapies, family services, client advocacy, and more. While many of these services are still available, the slowing of the HIV progression in the United States, as well as other factors, has contributed to a diminution in public interest and attention which may suggest that AIDS joining the ranks of other life-threatening illnesses that garner far fewer and less comprehensive resources.

For some HIV positive gay men, the attention, special care, and services they received begot a sense of entitlement, and a recent "fall from grace" into the realm of the ordinary, chronically ill person comes as a harsh narcissistic blow. For instance, one support group client admitted one day that he had decided to "boycott" a favorite restaurant of his when the restaurant ceased offering discounts to members of a community-based AIDS organization. To this client's mind, this change was understood as HIV/AIDS-based discrimination, rather than a more reality based understanding of economic constraints. One might ask why PWAS should be singled out to receive special treatment from others living with different terminal illnesses. Another client, in anticipation of the anniversary of September 11th, stated, "I'm sick of hearing about terrorism and September 11th, as far as I'm concerned it's all a big distraction away from HIV and AIDS." For a therapist, entitlement can be an uncomfortable issue to encounter, let alone address, in treatment with someone living with a life-threatening illness. Nonetheless, identifying the benefits that a client may have been afforded due to his HIV status, questioning and challenging a client's perspective with comparisons made to others dealing with illness, and providing empathic validation of the subsequent experience of change and loss may together offer useful restructuring interventions for clients struggling with the changing social status of HIV.

Apathy

While apathy in gay men living with HIV is often a symptom of depression, as in other chronic illnesses it is also an understandable outcome of living with years of ongoing uncertainty and unpredictability. Constant threats to life and physical well-being, body integrity and comfort, life goals and future plans, independence, privacy, autonomy and control is, at the very least, emotionally and psychologically wearing (Falvo, 1991). Imagine the impact of nearing death with no hope of survival, being offered a "miracle" in drugs that restored your health and functioning, engendering a hope for the future, and then having it all start to come crashing down. Or imagine facing the dilemma of being alive but not feeling well enough to do more than basically exist? How does one continue to maintain a positive outlook as well as a reason to live in light of these factors and others like them? In addition, many gay men living with HIV/AIDS have lost countless numbers of friends to this disease. The impact of continual loss and complicated bereavement can result in a state of impassivity (Summers, 1995). Therapists need to validate and empathize with a client's experience–to offer support in facing this existential crisis, and to help the client develop a sense of purpose. While individual therapy can help a client to stabilize his sense of self in the face of overwhelming instability and uncertainty, group therapy is particularly useful in helping alleviate the emotional distress underlying apathy by helping a client see that he is not alone in his suffering (Alfonso & Cohen, 1997; Goodheart, & Lansing, 1996; Kelly, 1998; Tunnell, 1994). In the support groups that I run, clients report finding strength in knowing that their problems are not unique, learning from others different ways to cope, as well as being inspired by the struggles and achievements that they observe.

CONFOUNDING FACTORS IN TREATMENT

There are many factors that can complicate psychotherapy with HIV positive gay men. These may include uncertainty with regard to the cause of a client's presenting condition (mental illness vs. medication side effects vs. chemical abuse); a preexisting history of emotional and psychological trauma that may include physical and/or sexual abuse and related sequelae such as a fragile sense of self, deep shame, or destructive behavior (compulsive sex, chemical abuse/dependence, putting oneself in risky situations, and a tenuous commitment to health); and characterological pathology.

As psychotherapists, we are trained to focus our attention on the emotional and psychological underpinnings of mental distress/illness. However, one of the clinical challenges therapists working with HIV positive gay men encounter, when trying to understand presenting symptoms and make a differential diagnosis, is distinguishing between psychosocial and biological causes (Budin, 1997; Tiamson, 2002). This challenge is most pronounced when presented with symptoms that are very similar to those seen in a depressive syndrome. Take, for instance, the case of Rodney:

> Rodney, a gay man in his early 40s, was referred for psychotherapy by his physician to address his depression. He had been living with HIV for several years and was in good physical condition. Since starting a regimen of HIV drugs, his blood work showed an undetected viral load, healthy number of T-cells, and no apparent

abnormalities. Rodney reported a period of low mood lasting over a year as well as profound fatigue, amotivation, anhedonia, and poor concentration. He had tried several different antidepressants and was receiving some benefit from the most recent one in addition to a stimulant to address his fatigue. After a consult with his physician seemed to rule out possible medical causes for his depressive symptoms, we began to explore possible underlying psychological issues. Treatment focused on conflictual familial relations, grief over the death of his mother, low self-esteem and difficulties with assertiveness. But psychotherapeutic gains were short-lived at best. Frustrated, Rodney suggested to his MD that perhaps his low mood was due to anemia, a condition common to people on HIV meds that had earlier been ruled out. Rodney insisted on further testing which revealed a mild case of anemia. Rodney was put on a drug that stimulates red blood cell production, which resulted in a marked improvement in mood and energy level. In addition, his self-esteem seemed restored and he no longer struggled with being assertive. We terminated treatment shortly thereafter.

This case illustrates a drug-mediated condition that presented primarily with mood and behavior symptoms that mimic a clinical depression. At different times during the course of treatment with Rodney, I felt dismayed with fleeting gains and wondered about the possibility of his resisting deeper therapeutic work. But the primary cause of Rodney's distress was physiological.

At other times what appears to be medication related is, in fact, psychologically determined. Consider the case of Louis:

Louis, a 45-year-old gay male, was a member of an HIV support group I co-facilitated as part of an Adult Day Health Center (ADHC) program for people with HIV/AIDS. In addition to multiple medical problems due to HIV/AIDS and obesity, he also had a long history of substance dependence in which he was ostensibly in recovery, as well as a mixed personality disorder. Louis would complain in group of profound fatigue, depression and bouts of anxiety. I consulted with his physician, psychiatrist and other caregivers to try to identify contributing factors. Group members and facilitators alike expressed deep concern to Louis regarding his condition, challenged him about possible drug/alcohol use (which he emphatically denied), and encouraged him to follow through with his medical appointments, to communicate with his physician and to seek further medical evaluation. It was not until Louis reluctantly went to the hospital emergency room because of chest pain that a drug screening revealed methamphetamine use. In response to treatment recommendations that included a chemical dependency (CD) treatment program, Louis became irate and belligerent and dropped out of the program.

This case, in particular, led to more stringent admission criteria at the ADHC when a history of a dual diagnosis of chemical dependency and a personality disorder is present. These clients are required to be actively involved in a CD program for a designated period of time before they are admitted. In addition, while unable to conduct a urine toxicology screen, we now frequently consult with the client's CD program where ongoing drug testing is done. While HIV/AIDS may indeed be a factor contributing to a client's distress, this case illustrates how many other psychological factors need to be disentangled in order to focus on what treatment issue is most paramount. It also highlights the current gap in services available to adequately treat dually diagnosed gay men living with HIV.

Other clients bring with them a history of emotional and psychological trauma that can play a part in their treatment in unexpected ways. Consider the case of Mark:

Mark, a gay man in his early 40s, began attending an HIV support group after being discharged from the hospital following meningitis. Individual psychotherapy with Mark revealed a history of ongoing sexual abuse. This experience, combined with an emotionally and physically abusive, alcoholic turned fundamentalist Christian father created a disturbingly traumatic early life for this man. Much of the early part of Mark's treatment involved an uncovering, experiencing and working through of the deep pain, sadness and anger that he had held at bay for so long. Toward the middle of treatment, Mark admitted that he had stopped taking his HIV meds for quite some time. He asserted a dogmatic, oppositional stance toward HIV/AIDS medication professing his belief that they would kill him as well as his disbelief that HIV causes AIDS. While an aspect of his assertion was not without merit, the intensity of his defensiveness and the secrecy surrounding his choice suggested the influence of deeper intrapsychic factors. I struggled with a sense of obligation to protect him from harm–that is, his decision to not take drugs could hasten his demise–while acknowledging and empathizing with the reality-based parts of his conflict. Reminding myself that his oppositional stance was rooted in unconscious conflict and was a defense against underlying pain, I was able to step back and take a more empathic stance. Without an argumentative partner in the dance of this dynamic, the noise that Mark was making was quieted and the further pain and distress regarding the emotional and psychological abuse was more readily available to him for further working through.

A focus on the particulars of Mark's medication argument, as well as the ramifications of his decision, would have overlooked the dynamic underpinnings and dissociative defenses that were fueling his behavior (Chu, 1992). By disentangling the strands of Mark's distress, he became aware of the different intrapsychic factors underlying his argument and was able to separate out: issues of power, control, self-destructiveness, identification with the aggressor, and a pattern of creating untenable situations in which he felt trapped with no where to turn. His intractable stance around HIV/AIDS drugs began to loosen and he was able to make decisions from a psychologically healthier place.

For Mark, conflict around HIV medication was a defense against deeper conflict and a recapitulation of intrapsychic issues and dynamics. A different example of how historical trauma can influence a client's current HIV/AIDS distress can be seen in the case of Tom, the gay man with a recent HIV seroconversion detailed earlier:

Tom's negative experience of himself in relationship to others preceded his HIV positive status and could be linked to his early childhood relationship with his mother. Tom's mother was characterized as an emotionally abusive woman whose behavior alternated between being affectionate to admonishing and condemning Tom. At the beginning of therapy, Tom's internal experience of himself was as "small, less than, afraid, and inadequate." This experience stood in contrast to his perception of most others as "big, better than, confident, and smart." His fears of being rejected because of HIV status fit into a characteristic pattern of seeing himself as flawed and not worthy. Attempts to challenge his feelings of being "damaged goods" due to HIV resulted in minimal change and deeper work on his *self-other* experience needed to be done. Tom's sense of self was restructured by helping him understand that this negative perception of himself was directly connected to an *other* (his mother) who was often rejecting. In addition, and essential to the work being fully effective, core affect, heretofore defensively suppressed or disavowed, was unearthed, experienced and worked through (Fosha, 2000). In our work together, Tom became comfortable with his adaptive anger toward his mother and, in doing so, began to see and experience himself in a more positive way. We were then able to address his HIV status as a separate issue.

In this case, HIV conflict or distress was not so much a defense, but rather the result of deep-seated negative feelings about the self based in historical childhood dynamics. As this case illustrates, work on HIV distress alone may not be adequate to alleviate client's struggles, and deeper intrapsychic conflicts need to be considered.

Lastly, severe mental health problems can, and do, color and complicate treatment for some in unexpected ways. Consider the case of Craig:

> Prior to his illness, Craig, a gay man in his late 30s, worked for a large corporation and prided himself on his success in his career as well as the company he kept. When he suffered a grand mal seizure and was hospitalized and subsequently diagnosed with AIDS, the facade that Craig had constructed to hide his homosexuality and a long history of anonymous sexual encounters was destroyed. The client's medical condition opened a window which revealed a narcissistic personality disorder marked by a fragile sense of self, deep-seated guilt, shame and rage, and a desperate longing for approval. Individual and group therapy tried to help the client see his parents more realistically and begin to acknowledge and experience his conflicted feelings toward them as well as develop compassion toward himself and others. Craig seemed to be making progress, but group members and facilitators were alarmed when Craig admitted beginning to engage in risky, violent sexual encounters. The group tried to break through his defensive stance, but his denial of danger was intractable. Treatment was cut short when Craig was found dead in his home, apparently the victim of a sexual encounter gone awry.

Craig's behavior and condition was dramatically influenced by character pathology that far overshadowed his HIV-related issues. For men who were emotionally and psychology impaired prior to HIV infection, particularly those with characterological impairment, psychotherapy can be slow going with minimal change over long periods of time. In Craig's case, great efforts had been made to address Craig's self-destructive behavior by his individual psychotherapist, the Day Health staff, his case manager and his physician. In the aftermath of Craig's death, many of those involved in his care struggled with negotiating issues of responsibility and blame, a common challenge when working with seriously wounded clients. While anger at clients who reject essential help can be an understandable reaction for the clinician, it is essential to keep in mind that the maladaptive behavioral patterns of such clients are usually unconsciously motivated and out of reach of conscious engagement. This awareness can be invaluable in helping to navigate an often difficult and disturbing terrain without further shaming the patient.

THERAPIST FACTORS

By now it should be clear that psychotherapy with HIVpositive gay men has particular challenges for both the client and therapist alike. In addition to the different factors already discussed, therapists doing this work are subject to countertransferential phenomena that are similar to those encountered in psychotherapy with clients with other chronic, life-threatening illnesses. For instance, anxieties around loss, death, vulnerability and uncertainty are all common (Goodheart & Lansing, 1996). As HIV/AIDS still poses a threat to life, therapists need to be able to facilitate work that includes facing the possibility of death, grappling with feelings about death, and preparing to die. In addition to death, anxiety around loss is possible as clients' losses of functioning, employment and social status can call to the therapist's mind his or her own personal losses. It is difficult for therapists to effectively help a client face these issues and the attendant fears and feelings without addressing their own feelings regarding both mortality and loss. When addressed, these feelings can be used therapeutically to enhance the treatment; when not, they can lead to disengagement, numbness and burnout (Gabriel, 1996). To avoid burnout when dealing with issues of death, grief and loss, therapists can seek professional supervision and consultation, talk with and seek support from colleagues, establish a work/life balance and find ways to nurture and care for the self.

For the therapist, emotional openness to deep affective states enables us to be present for our clients in a real way and to be "alive" and authentic in our work (Fosha, 2000). By making space for the experiences of loss, grief and pain that is inevitably a part of psychotherapy, clients are enabled to ride the wave of their adaptive feelings toward a healthy place of acceptance and peace. A therapist's willingness to go on this journey with the client is key to lessening the emotional burden and undoing a sense of aloneness.

Lastly, as mentioned earlier, an issue unique to HIV/AIDS has to do with the disease being transmitted sexually. It is not uncommon for fears of HIV infection to come up for therapists working with HIV positive gay men as we are human beings who are also sexual. For therapists who are also gay men, the work is rife with opportunities for overidentification with the client. For those therapists who are also HIV positive, fears around the course of illness that may be similar to or different from the client are also likely. Having a clear and realistic sense of one's own health status and level of risk can help to diminish anxieties and allow therapists to navigate these sometimes turbulent and murky waters. For those therapists who may not be comfortable with their own health status and/or sexual risk taking, awareness alone may not be sufficient in assuaging anxiety; personal psychotherapy may be indicated should these issues continue to be a source of significant conflict.

CONCLUSION

If history is any indication of what is yet to come, we can anticipate continued changes in the kinds of struggles HIV positive gay men will encounter. As clinicians working with this population, our knowledge and understanding of HIV/AIDS processes and treatments, as well as the psychosocial stressors of chronic illnesses in general, needs to stay current. Our understanding of the varied challenges each client is facing, an awareness and attunement to the multitude of factors that can complicate treatment, our willingness to be emotionally open, and our ability to be flexible in our therapeutic approach will all go a long way toward helping us effectively meet the needs of our clients.

REFERENCES

Alfonso, C. A. & Cohen, M. A. (1997). The role of group therapy in the care of person with AIDS. *Journal of the American Academy of Psychoanalysis, 25*(4), 623-638.

Brashers, D. E., Neidig. J. L., Cardillo, L. W.; Dobbs, L. K., Russell, J. A., Haas, S. M. (1999). "In an important way, I did die": Uncertainty and renewal in persons living with HIV or AIDS, *AIDS Care, 11*(2), 201-219.

Buckingham, S. L. & Van Gorp, W. G. (1999). HIV-associated cognitive/motor complex: Early detection, diagnosis, and intervention. In M. Shernoff (Ed.), *AIDS and mental health practice: Clinical and policy issues* (pp. 285-306). New York: The Haworth Press, Inc.

Budin, J. (1997). Understanding neuropsychiatric and psychological symptoms in the context of HIV illness. In L.A. Wicks (Ed.), *Psychotherapy and AIDS: The human dimension* (pp. 53-77). Washington, DC: Taylor & Francis.

Chu, J. A. (1992). The therapeutic roller coaster: Dilemmas in the treatment of childhood abuse survivors. *Journal of Psychotherapy Practice and Research, 1*(4), 351-370.

Falvo, D. R. (1991). *Medical and psychosocial aspects of chronic illness and disability*. Gaithersburg, MD: Aspen.

Farber, E. W. & McDaniel, J. S. (1999). Assessment and psychotherapy practice implications of new combination antiviral therapies for HIV disease. *Professional Psychology: Research and Practice, 30*(2), 173-179.

Fosha, D. (2000). *The transforming power of affect: A model for accelerated change*. New York, NY: Basic Books.

Gabriel, M. A. (1996). *Aids trauma and support group therapy: Mutual aid, empowerment and connection*. New York, NY: The Free Press.

Goodheart, C. D. & Lansing, M. H. (1996). *Treating people with chronic disease: A psychological guide*. Washington, D.C.: American Psychological Association.

Green, J. & Sherr, L. (1989). Dying, bereavement and loss. In J. Green & A. McCreaner (Eds.), *Counseling in HIV infection and AIDS* (pp. 207-223). Cambridge, MA: Blackwell Scientific Publications, Inc..

Kelly, J. A. (1998). Group psychotherapy for persons with HIV and AIDS related illnesses. *International Journal of Group Psychotherapy, 48*(2), 143-162.

National Institute of Allergy and Infectious Diseases (2002). Fact Sheet. National Institute of Health. NIAID Website.

Rabkin, J. G., Ferrando, S. J., VanGorp, W., Rieppi, R., McElhiney, M., & Sewell, M. (2000). Relationships among apathy, depression, and cognitive impairment in HIV/AIDS. *Journal of Neuropsychiatry and Clinical Neuroscience, 12*, 451-457.

Stephenson, J. (2002). Sobering levels of drug resistant HIV found. *Journal of the American Medical Association, 287*, 6.

Summers, J. (1995). Psychiatric morbidity associated with AIDS-related grief resolution. *Journal of Nervous and Mental Disease, 183*(6), 384-389.

Tiamson, M. L. (2002). Challenges in the management of the HIV patient in the third decade of AIDS. *Psychiatric Quarterly, 73*(1), 51-58.

Tunnell, G. (1994). Special issues in group psychotherapy for gay men with AIDS. In S. A. Caldwell, R. A. Burnham, & M. Forstein (Eds.), *Therapists on the frontline: Psychotherapy with gay men in the age of AIDS* (pp. 237-254). Washington, DC: American Psychiatric Press.

Weiss, J. J. (1997). Psychotherapy with HIV-positive gay men: A psychodynamic perspective. *American Journal of Psychotherapy, 51*, 1, 31-44.

Yalom, I. D. (1985). *The theory and practice of group psychotherapy (3rd edition)*. New York: Basic Books.

Zuger, A. (2002, July 16). Beyond temporary 'miracles.' *The New York Times*, p. F5.

Resistance and Resilience:
The Untold Story of Gay Men Aging
with Chronic Illnesses

John Genke

SUMMARY. Few studies have looked at the aging process in terms of sexual orientation, and none have focused on the role that chronic health concerns play in this relationship. This article begins a more comprehensive theoretical exploration of the connection between aging, chronic illness, and sexual orientation. The author employs his practice experiences as a social worker for chronically ill and aging gay men to highlight key issues for this population, including resilience in the face of crises; mistrust of the mainstream medical and social service institutions; and internally and externally located obstacles to receiving effective medical and psychosocial care. Effective intervention strategies to serve this population are presented. *[Article copies available for a fee from The Haworth Document Delivery Service: 1-800-HAWORTH. E-mail address: <docdelivery@haworthpress.com> Website: <http://www.HaworthPress.com> © 2004 by The Haworth Press, Inc. All rights reserved.]*

John Genke, MSW, CSW, is Senior Social Worker, Senior Action in a Gay Environment (SAGE), 305 Seventh Avenue, 16th Floor, New York, NY 10001 (E-mail: sageusa@aol.com or johngenke@yahoo.com).

The author wishes to acknowledge the assistance of Benjamin Lipton, the editor of this volume, in preparing this article for publication.

[Haworth co-indexing entry note]: "Resistance and Resilience: The Untold Story of Gay Men Aging with Chronic Illnesses." Genke, John. Co-published simultaneously in *Journal of Gay & Lesbian Social Services* (Harrington Park Press, an imprint of The Haworth Press, Inc.) Vol. 17, No. 2, 2004, pp. 81-95; and: *Gay Men Living with Chronic Illnesses and Disabilities: From Crisis to Crossroads* (ed: Benjamin Lipton) Harrington Park Press, an imprint of The Haworth Press, Inc., 2004, pp. 81-95. Single or multiple copies of this article are available for a fee from The Haworth Document Delivery Service [1-800-HAWORTH, 9:00 a.m. - 5:00 p.m. (EST). E-mail address: docdelivery@haworthpress.com].

Digital Object Identifier: 10.1300/J041v17n02_05

KEYWORDS. Coming out, crisis competence, resilience, passing, gay, gerontology, invisibility, cultural imperialism, friendly visitor, home care

"Don't get old, it's terrible!" is the oft-repeated refrain of many of the clients at Senior Action in a Gay Environment (SAGE) in New York City. These clients are people 60 years of age and older who identify, either explicitly or tacitly, as lesbian, gay, bisexual, or transgendered. (LGBT People Living with HIV/AIDS become eligible for SAGE's social services at age 50.) In keeping with the theme of this volume, this article will focus specifically on SAGE's male clients.

So what are these men talking about when they utter the above lament? It can be said with certainty that they are not referring to their sexual orientation. The stereotype of the lonely, bitter, old "queen" has been debunked in most of the literature on gay aging to emerge in the 30-odd years since Stonewall (Wahler & Gabbay, 1997). In fact, as this article will illustrate, even individuals who apparently conform to such a stereotype, upon closer examination often reveal hidden reservoirs of courage and resiliency, born out of their early, unavoidable struggle with the "coming out" process.

It is argued that successfully negotiating the coming out process gives gay men a certain advantage over their straight counterparts because gay men are forced to cope with stigma and loss at a much earlier age (Kooden, 1997; Quam & Whitford, 1992; Pope and Schultz, 1991; Kimmel, 1978). Kimmel (1978) named this dynamic "crisis competence" (p.117). Both Kooden (1997) and D'Augelli (1994) suggest that crisis competence which results from negotiating the coming out process provides gay men with the basis for addressing all future life crises, including those connected to aging. Wahler and Gabbay (1997) indicate that relative satisfaction in terms of aging hinges upon the gay man, at the very least, being out to himself. This may account for some of the resiliency noted above in otherwise closeted individuals.

Most often, SAGE clients fall somewhere in the mid-range of a three-part spectrum of gay identity formation as conceptualized by Friend (in Kooden, 1997). At one end is the aforementioned stereotype steeped in internalized homophobia (the lonely, bitter, self-hating "queen"); at the opposite pole is the self-accepting, self-affirming gay man. Between the two poles reside those whom Friend describes as "passing": gay men who have achieved conditional acceptance of their sexual orientation, but who remain closeted in some portion of their lives (where they "pass" as straight), and maintain a more or less marginal connection with the gay community. The majority of SAGE's clients fall into this midrange category, and it is these men whose situations this article will address.

GAY GERONTOLOGY

As Wahler and Gabbay (1997) point out, the study of gay gerontology is a recent phenomenon, currently spanning little more than three decades and comprising a miniscule body of work. At the time of their review, they found only 58 empirically based studies on the subject. Woolf (1998) notes that most of this research has focused on people 40 years of age and older with few studies conducted solely on individuals over 60. Most of these studies focus on "breaking down the negative myths surrounding older gay men" (Wahler & Gabbay, 1997, p. 5). There appears to be nothing in the literature specifically addressing the relationship between sexual orientation and the chronic health conditions associated with aging. This scarcity of information, both in scope and in content, creates a serious knowledge gap, not only in terms of gay aging, but also in terms of aging in general. As Kooden (1997) points out, "traditional developmental theory is based on an assumption of heterosexuality" (p. 22). Therefore, the developmental tasks necessary for gay men to successfully negotiate the passages, first into midlife and then into old age, with its incumbent physical deterioration, remain virtually unexplored and unarticulated. Yet it is apparent that many gay men have to some degree successfully negotiated these transitions despite the fact that they do not conform to accepted, heterosexually based developmental patterns, indicating the unique strengths and creative coping strategies of older gay men. Information culled from empirical studies of these special competencies would very likely benefit the aging population in general (Kooden, 1997; Wahler & Gabbay, 1997).

In this article, the author will draw from his experiences working with aging gay men at SAGE to illustrate some of the ways these men are dealing with their chronic health concerns, and how their histories as gay men may affect their coping strategies. The article will also examine some of the interventions SAGE has found particularly helpful in assisting its clients. Additionally, some of the obstacles to providing this assistance will be identified. Hopefully, this preliminary exploration will pave the way for the more extensive empirical research needed to create a healthier picture of aging for all gays and, by extension, for the aging population in general. It must be noted that the majority of SAGE's population is white, educated, middle class, and urban. This demographic profile has been true for the vast majority of empirical studies of the LGBT population (Kooden, 1997; Wahler & Gabbay, 1997). It should therefore be kept in mind that the information presented herein is specific to a very small group of aging gay men.

AGING, LOSS, AND THE IMPACT OF AIDS

The lament from the beginning of this article ("Don't get old, it's terrible!") usually refers most immediately to the physical aches, pains and decreases in functioning that are brought on by chronic conditions associated with aging: heart disease, arthritis, emphysema, diabetes, glaucoma, and hearing loss, to name but a few of the many things that also lead some SAGE clients to lament, "I never thought would happen to me." On a deep level, these admonitions against aging refer to physical and emotional losses that declines in health bring on. These losses include those of freedom and autonomy that these individuals had previously enjoyed, as well as the social roles that gave them purpose and direction. In a very real and frightening sense, the aging processes of these men become, in their own minds and in the minds of a terrified ageist society at large, fused and thus confused with disease. Their sense of themselves as they once were is shattered. In addition to personal declines in functioning, the lament includes absences of friends, partners, parents, and siblings–those anchors of their social and historical context–lost through estrangement, relocation, their own ill health, or death.

Interestingly, all this begins to sound like what young gay men experienced at the height of the AIDS epidemic before the advent of combination therapy in the mid-nineties: the sense of incredulity, the suffering and loss, and the identification with disease. There is an important difference, however, between what those men went through and what gay men aging with chronic illnesses experience. That difference is the tremendous amount of support that gay men living with AIDS received from the gay community, fueled by a collective anger at the injustice being done them, as opposed to the indifference that ill and aging gay men have almost always encountered from the very same community. Ironically, many of the men who are now experiencing this indifference were at the forefront of the fight against AIDS. Many of these men lost whole friendship networks to that disease. A number of them are themselves living with HIV. Now that the ardor of AIDS activism in the community has cooled, they are left to wonder how they survived and why. Older gay men living with HIV may be particularly affected by this dynamic. Harley, a 63-year-old gay man living with the virus put it this way:

> I have had long relationships, 20 years or more, with men who were dying, and you never shake that. It never leaves you . . . I still remember them. I know the month they died. It's this terrible lone-liness from all the people you knew that are gone, and watching people around you . . . die. And then you get this feeling of guilt, of why am I still here? (*Newsline*, 1996, p. 12)

Surprisingly, my experience with SAGE clients suggests that there is little bitterness expressed about the indifference of gay communities to them. The sentiment is more of resignation. Perhaps the loss of so many peers, a tremendous portion of a whole generation, and the ensuing sur-vivor guilt lowers expectations. Internalized ageism may also be a fac-tor. Several men have remarked that they never wanted to be around old gay men when they were young, so why should they expect younger gay men to feel differently now. The crisis competence referred to earlier may be another factor at work here. The image comes to mind, particu-larly in regard to older men living with HIV, of a group huddled bravely and stoically on an ice floe that is disappearing out to sea.

DOUBLE INVISIBILITY

When introduced to the services of SAGE, non-gay social service professionals as well as lay people often will want to know what distin-guishes the needs of aging gays from those of the old in general. Why is SAGE a necessary organization? While this inquiry is usually prompted by genuine interest, the very asking of the question reveals the heterosexist as-sumptions that inform such inquiry. In fact, there is general agreement that most aging adults, gay or straight, face the same major concerns, and they mostly involve loss. These concerns are, as Quam and Whitford (1992) put it, "loneliness, health, and income" (p. 373). Underlying these common concerns is the stigma attached to aging. Just as a heterosexist society discriminates against gay people, so an ageist soci-ety discriminates against old people (Cahill et al., 2000). Witness the lack of positive terms for old people in our language and the plethora of derogatory ones: "geezer," "fogey," "dirty old man," "old fart," etc. (Genke, 2000; Engle, 1998). Expressions such as "You don't look your age" and the reluctance to talk about age in general reinforce this devalued status, as does the enduring cultural obsession with procedures that inhibit looking old, such as plastic surgery, botox injections, and "anti-ageing" unguents. Systemically across the culture, the old are devalued, excluded and discriminated against. And this is perhaps even more the case for the older gay man residing in the youth-obsessed gay subculture (Cahill et al., 2000). As with homophobia, even for the most "self-actualized" gay men, the negative messages of ageism are unavoidably internalized not only by the young, but also by the old.

MARGINALIZATION

In her book *Justice and the Politics of Difference*, Young (1990) identifies what she labels "Five Faces of Oppression." One of those faces she terms "marginalization." Among those who experience this face of oppression are the old. Young describes marginalization as "perhaps the most dangerous [face of oppression because] a whole category of people is expelled from useful participation in social life [and thus faces] potential extermination" (p. 53) (at least, the author would add, in a metaphorical sense). "Uselessness, boredom, and lack of self-respect" (p. 55) constitute the internalized feelings Young identifies as being induced by this form of oppression. When the old speak of feeling "invisible," it is this sense of marginalization, of metaphorical extermination, that they are describing. When old gay people speak of feeling "invisible," their sense of marginalization reawakens and reinforces existing stigma from an early age when they first identified and/or were identified with homosexuality. Moreover, ageism denies, or at least conceals, the sexuality of the old (Genke, 2000; Huff, 1998). Thus, older gay men are not only rendered invisible because they are old, but also because as desexualized older people, their sexual orientation loses meaning within ageist culture.

AGEIST OPPRESSION WITHIN GAY COMMUNITIES

Sadly, this invisibility holds true, perhaps especially, in gay communities, where ageism may be even more pronounced. Cahill et al. (2000) cite "beauty standards that privilege youth" (p.18), whose sense of meaning and value is inextricably linked to "physical attractiveness and desirability" (p.18), as an obvious manifestation of this phenomenon. Berger (1982) notes young gay men who worry that they are "over the hill" as early as age thirty. Cahill et al. (2000) go on to describe other more subtle manifestations of ageism in the gay community (and hence, perhaps more damaging to the self-concept of older gays). They point out that community discussions exclude old people and that senior issues are conspicuously absent from the mainstream LGBT political agenda. Furthermore, they assert that the ageism in the gay community is structural: gay organizations and institutions are age-segregated, outreach to the old is nonexistent (e.g., the lack of senior discounts to gay events), and the achievements of gay elders are rarely honored. With the exception of LBGT religious communities, few gay organizations are intentionally intergenerational.

It should be noted here that in the same way old people may collude in their own invisibility via their internalized ageism, old gay people may collude in their double invisibility via their internalized homophobia and ageism; this will hold true even if they have been relatively out in their younger years. Those who work with older gay men posit that old gay men tend to retreat back into the closet when they need to access mainstream service providers (Altman, 1999). The same retreat often occurs when they come in contact with heterosexual old people in senior centers and the like. In these settings, internalized homophobia is linked to an expectation of prejudice, since homophobia is generally more prevalent among older generations in this country, who have internalized the same homophobic messages as their peers, than it is in the population as a whole (Cahill et al., 2000).

CULTURAL IMPERIALISM

Young (1990) includes what she labels "cultural imperialism" among the Five Faces of Oppression discussed earlier (p. 58). The heterosexist culture which gives rise to homophobia is a vivid example of this phenomenon. In cultural imperialism, the dominant cultural group (e.g., heterosexuals) imposes on the oppressed group (e.g., gays) its experience and interpretation of social life while rendering the oppressed group's particular perspective invisible and at the same time stereotyping that group and marking it out as the Other.

> Those living under cultural imperialism find themselves defined from the outside, positioned, placed, by a network of dominant meanings they experience as arising from elsewhere, from those with whom they do not identify and who do not identify with them. (Young, p. 59)

Young (1990) invokes the words of W.E.B. Du Bois to describe the "double consciousness" that results from this imperialism. Even as the oppressed group is being negatively stereotyped by the dominant culture and is itself internalizing those negative images, it is also creating and sustaining its own affirmative culture that allows its members to develop a sense of positive identity. One example of this double consciousness is manifested in the phenomenon of "camp," with which much of older gay culture is imbued. As Clark (1987) suggests, by enacting the effeminate stereotype, gay men appear to appease the dominant group even while enjoying among themselves the knowledge that they are "flaunt[ing] the lie of the stereotype in the face of the bigot" (p. 99).

Moreover, the cultural imperialism imposed on gay men by a heterosexist society seems to parallel that which an ageist gay community imposes upon its senior members. Within gay cultures, young gay men may be seen as comprising a dominant group who oppress, both actively and by unconscious omission, old gay men. This situation implies multiple layers of invisibility for old gay men: first as old within the larger society, second as old and gay within the larger society, third as gay within the aging community, and fourth as old within the gay community. If you add to the mix such factors as ethnicity, socioeconomic class, geographical situation, and chronic health concerns, then untangling the web of invisibility and shedding light on the experience and needs of this population confronts service providers with significant challenges.

INTERVENTION STRATEGIES: ONE AGENCY'S RESPONSE

SAGE's mission is to provide a place where old LGBT people can feel supported, embraced and celebrated (Altman, 1999). Establishing, reestablishing, or maintaining a connection to the LGBT community by creating a sense of a surrogate family is a vital component of this mission. Depending upon the needs and circumstances of a particular client, interventions to achieve this goal can take various forms. For those gay men who have struggled most of their lives with unresolved issues around sexual identity, calling upon SAGE is often their first contact with a gay-identified organization, so that for SAGE to simply exist and be available is already a form of intervention. For most men, direct contact with SAGE results from a personal crisis, often health related: the need for home care, bereavement counseling, or access to entitlements.

Frequently, contact also is initiated by informed service providers who refer their clients to the agency. Other times, friends and even family members will do the contacting.

In addition to gay affirmative case management and clinical services, SAGE offers a wide range of socialization opportunities, including group activities, socials, activism, and volunteer options. Unlike SAGE social services, which are limited to people age 60 and above, socialization opportunities welcome adults of all ages, opening the door to potential intergenerational interaction. Empirical data has shown that integration into the gay community through active participation in social activities leads to greater life satisfaction for gay people. Individuals become more self-accepting, less depressed, and less fearful of aging (Quam & Whitford, 1992; Berger, 1982). As Vaillant (in Lambert, 2001) describes in *Aging Well*, his account of Harvard University's landmark longitudinal study on adult development, "Feeling safe, secure, and 'held' allows us to use more mature defenses" (p. 99). This would appear to hold true even for gay men of advanced age with little previous connection to the community.

Friendly visiting is one of the most significant interventions that SAGE provides. Volunteers are matched, according to interests and compatibility, with homebound or semi-homebound clients who lack social supports such as family or available friends. These volunteers agree to visit their "friends-at-home" weekly for an hour or two as well as to check in weekly by phone. If the client is ambulatory, the visitor can go out with him to eat, see a movie, attend a SAGE event, or just sit in the park and talk. Each summer, SAGE sponsors a picnic where friends and their visitors can meet and celebrate together. Often, if he is truly homebound, this is the only time the friend-at-home has the opportunity to attend an outside event. SAGE provides the transportation, and the staff and members of the board host the event along with the volunteers.

One of the important benefits of the friendly visitor program is the opportunity it provides for intergenerational contact and the resultant generativity that often ensues. The visitors are usually a generation or two removed from the friend they visit. They speak of how they are changed and affected by the work they do. Old, homebound gay men are presented with an opportunity to find meaning and purpose in this stage of life, and younger volunteers become the bearers of gay history in the same way families of origin carry their members' stories forward.

For those with more specific, concrete service needs, SAGE's Lend-A-Hand program provides volunteers on an ad hoc basis to help clients with more practical matters. This may include escorting someone to a medical appointment, shopping, delivering a package, putting up a shelf, or installing a computer program, the kinds of things that family members or friends might do for their older relatives.

CASE EXAMPLE

Val was a closeted, 82-year-old gay man when he contacted SAGE. He was referred to SAGE by his psychotherapist, who had recommended increased socialization. Val was likable but rather reserved. He had resided in his spartan, meticulously neat walk-up apartment in the far reaches of one of the boroughs of New York City for more than forty years. Before retirement, he had done white collar work for an institution in Manhattan and was financially comfortable. Since the death of his beloved sister, he was estranged from his other siblings and their families and had been living an increasingly lonely and isolated existence. It was clear that his poor self-image contributed to this estrangement. He was easily hurt and built up strong and bitter resentments against his family for what he perceived as slights and neglect. Though he had never married a woman to "pass," as many gay men of his generation had done, he had also never come out to his family or work associates. His gay contacts were limited to anonymous sexual encounters in men's rooms and bars.

He was receptive to a home visit by the SAGE worker, and quickly agreed to accept a friendly visitor on a trial basis. Fortunately, there was a volunteer in Val's neighborhood, a stroke of unusual luck for this remote location. The visitor was a warm and intelligent retired professional in his early sixties who provided the first open relationship Val had ever experienced with another gay man. Eventually, as their relationship grew, Val dared to venture to a few SAGE events at the LGBT Community Center in Manhattan. This was an act of courage for someone so closeted and an indication of the possibility of growth and change even in old age. That Val had sought out psychotherapy as this late stage in his life, even before contacting SAGE, also testifies to his resilience.

It became apparent to the worker during a reassessment visit a few months later that Val could use some home care services. His heart was deteriorating and a pacemaker had been installed.

He had blacked out and fallen several times. He was having increasing difficulty negotiating the stairs to his apartment. Shopping in his neighborhood was several blocks away. However, admitting that he was proud and stubborn, he refused all suggestions of home care.

When he left a message some time later with his SAGE social worker suggesting it was time to "consider" home care, it was clear to his provider that things had taken a serious turn. Unable to reach him, the social worker learned, with the help of the friendly visitor, that Val had been admitted to the hospital. He was clearly delusional. He told the social worker during a hospital visit that he had returned home briefly a couple of days before (which was impossible, given his physical condition), where he had discovered his apartment robbed and ransacked. Returning to the hospital, he said he found a note on his pillow telling him to leave, that "his kind" weren't wanted there. He heard a voice whispering to him, "We know you're gay!" The social worker was able to help Val acknowledge that most likely he had imagined these experiences, and that he was very scared. During this visit, he gave the social worker permission to reveal to the hospital personnel his relationship to SAGE. (Many SAGE clients do not want to be associated with a gay agency, so SAGE has an alternate name–which the worker had been using–to assure confidentiality.) To the SAGE worker, this represented a courageous act of coming out.

Val died a few days later. It would appear that the "holding" presence of a gay-identified social service agency in the person of a trusted social worker and a supportive gay volunteer had a lot to do with Val's self-disclosure in the hospital. Certainly the quality of his last few years of life improved by the connection to the gay community, limited as it was, that SAGE provided him.

According to Friend's (1991) model of sexual identity formation among older gay people referred to earlier in this article, Val would fall into the lower end of the category of "passing." Though he did not marry, he lived a double life. He did not come out to friends or family; he limited his sexual life to anonymous secret encounters; and did not want the SAGE worker to reveal his association with him to other providers. His paranoid delusions in the hospital, while indeterminate in terms of a cause, vividly convey the strong hold that internalized homophobia had on Val.

While most of the clients at SAGE fall into this intermediate category of "passing" on the continuum of disclosure of sexual orientation, this does not mean that these men are without self-acceptance or gay affirmative sentiments. How one integrates a gay identity and manages disclosure is a complex, nonlinear, fluid process. Note that Val sought out psychotherapy at an advanced age and opened his door to SAGE services, hardly a template of despair. For many pre-Stonewall gay men, "passing" was a necessary and positive approach to managing stigma (Adelman, 1991). To be out unconditionally was not safe. The social message was clear: Sex between men was a criminal act; it was, according to mental health professionals, both abnormal and perverse; and mainstream religion saw it as sinful and worthy of hellfire (Altman, 1999; Kochman, 1997). Therefore, creating their own ways of living within safe limits, either as single gay men or as gay men in relationships, was a means of self-preservation. As Adelman (1991) puts it: ". . . the closets of the pre-Stonewall era provided comfort in a hostile environment by allowing one to have a positive image" (p. 30).

The legacy of passing can manifest in complex ways among aging gay men. For example, one of the major obstacles the author faces in working with aging gay men with chronic health conditions is their refusal to accept needed home care. Because old gay people like Val are more likely to live alone and have no informal caregiver to turn to (Cahill et al., 2000), this poses a real danger of self-neglect. In fact, a disproportionate number of neglect cases are composed of old gay people (Cook-Daniels, 2001). The self-reliance which had served gay men like Val well in the past as a survival mechanism becomes in the present a double-edged sword; It is both a strength and an obstacle to receiving necessary assistance.

Objections to accepting care can range from not being able to afford it, as in the cases of those ineligible for insurance benefits or entitlements, or in cases of those like Val who can afford it, to denial of need. Underlying these objections are the aforementioned value of self-reliance along with the not unfounded fear of discrimination. There are no home care agencies in New York City dedicated to caring for old gay people, and few provide LGBT sensitivity training to their workers (Altman, 1999). Consequently, when homecare is accessed, although the client's health status and functioning may improve, the quality of that client's life often deteriorates. One of the reasons for this is a feeling of being held prisoner in one's own home by once again having to pass as straight. We find that gay couples often tell health care providers that their partner is their "cousin" or "stepbrother." In this way, the absence of gay affirmative care reinforces internalized homophobia and impairs psychosocial health.

CONCLUSION

As they age, most people develop chronic health conditions of some kind. Some of these conditions can be relatively benign and easily manageable, while others are severe and traumatic. People living with chronic illnesses may become more dependent on health care, government and social service institutions. They need more medical attention; they are hospitalized; they go to rehabilitation in skilled nursing facilities; they need home care; and they may need to apply for housing and/or health care benefits. For aging gay men, these institutions still symbolize the cultural imperialism of the heterosexist establishment. Accessing services can feel threatening and reawaken fears of discrimination experienced earlier in their lives. If older gay men have not successfully come to terms with their sexual identities, then they may avoid seeking the care that they need and fall into self-neglect and isolation, exacerbated by their identification with the ageist attitudes that society imposes.

Even as social service providers advocate for and with this population to access appropriate assistance and support, it is important to keep in mind the often discounted courage and resilience older gay men have shown all their lives in the face of institutionalized homophobia. It is equally important to notice these same strengths as older gay men cope, again in often not-so-apparent ways, with institutionalized ageism. Without this awareness, workers can lose sight of the full humanity of their clients, whose quality of life and self-determinism may then be jeopardized.

For their physical, mental and spiritual health, gay men aging with chronic health issues need to be helped to connect physically and emotionally to the gay community. SAGE has been engaged in just such work for 25 years, but it is able to serve only a fraction of the aging gay population. There appear to be no other organizations offering the range of social services, socialization opportunities, education and advocacy that SAGE provides. Moreover, SAGE's expertise has been gained serving a predominantly white, urban, middle-class population, and most of the empirical research in gay gerontology, scant as it is, has been done on this same cohort. SAGE has just begun the work of building a relationship with communities of color. While this holds enormous promise, the lack of culturally competent research in this domain presents SAGE, and indeed the entire LGBT community, with enormous challenges which must be met if social justice is to be served.

As baby boomers age, the need to address the health care and well-being of older gay men is being felt all over the country and all over the world. Their numbers and needs will only increase in the coming decades. While needs will change along with the socio-historic perspectives of clients, ageism and homophobia, it seems, will remain as formidable obstacles for the foreseeable future. Thus, if gay men are to have the rich old age they deserve, they will require services that will help them to feel "safe, secure, and 'held' " (Lambert, 2001, p. 99) and to live meaningfully and productively. These services need to be developed from and supported by cogent empirical research. Such research will have enormous ramifications on the whole field of gerontology as the unique coping styles and strategies of a long-ignored population are identified and explored for the greater good of all old people now and in years to come.

REFERENCES

Adelman, M. A. (1991). Stigma, gay lifestyles, and adjustment to aging: A study of later-life gay men and lesbians. *Journal of Homosexuality, 20*(3-4), 7-32.

Altman, C. (1999). Gay and lesbian seniors: Unique challenges of coming out in later life. *Siecus Report, 27*(3), 14-17.

Berger, R. (1982). The unseen minority: Older gays and lesbians. *Social Work, 27,* 236-242.

Cahill, S., South, K., & Spade, J. (2000). *Outing age. Public policy issues affecting gay, lesbian, bisexual and transgender elders.* The Policy Institute of the National Gay and Lesbian Task Force.

Clark, D. (1987). *Loving someone gay, revised and updated.* Berkeley, CA: Celestial Arts.

Cook-Daniels, L. (1997). Lesbian, gay male, bisexual and transgendered elders: Elder abuse and neglect issues. *Journal of Elder Abuse and Neglect, 9*(2), 35-49.

D'Augelli, A. (1994). Lesbian and gay development: Steps toward an analysis of lesbian's and gay men's lives. In B. Greene and G. Herek (Eds.), *Psychological perspectives on lesbian & gay issues: Vol. 1. Lesbian & gay psychology: Theory, research and clinical applications* (pp. 118-132). Thousand Oaks, CA: Sage.

Engle, L. (1998). Old AIDS. *Body Positive, 11*(1), 14-21.

Friend, R. A. (1991). Older lesbian and gay people: A theory of successful aging. In J. A. Lee (Ed.), *Gay midlife and maturity* (pp. 99-118). New York: Harrington Park Press.

Genke, J. (2000). HIV/AIDS and older adults: The invisible ten percent. *The Journal of Long Term Home Health Care*, *2*(3), 196-205.

Huff, C. (1998). The age of ignorance. *POZ*, *12*, 59-63.

Kimmel, D. C. (1978). Adult development and aging: A gay perspective. *Journal of Social Issues*, *34*, 113-130.

Kochman, A. (1997). Gay and lesbian elderly: Historical overview and implications for social work practice. *Journal of Gay and Lesbian Social Services*, *6*(1), 1-10.

Kooden, H. (1997). Successful aging in the middle-aged gay man: A contribution to developmental theory. *Journal of Gay and Lesbian Social Services*, *6*(3), 21-43.

Lambert, C. (2001). The talent for aging well. *Harvard Magazine*, *103*(3-4), 45-47, 99.

Newsline (1996). AIDS and the aging. January, 7-17.

Pope, M., & Schultz, R. (1991). Sexual attitudes and behavior in midlife and aging homosexual males. In A. Lee (Ed.), *Gay midlife and maturity* (pp. 169-177). New York: Harrington Park Press.

Quam, J. K., & Whitford, G. S. (1992). Adaptation and age-related expectations of older gay and lesbian adults. *The Gerontologist*, *32*(3), 367-374.

Wahler, J., & Gabbay, S. G. (1997). Gay male aging: A review of the literature. *Journal of Gay and Lesbian Social Services*, *6*(3), 1-20.

Woolf, L. M. (1998). Gay and lesbian aging. Webster University Website, 1-4.

Young, I. M. (1990). *Justice and the politics of difference*. Princeton University Press.

The Impact of a Non-HIV Chronic Illness on Professional Practice: Personal and Professional Considerations of a Psychotherapist

Charles P. Isola

SUMMARY. This article discusses how a non-HIV-related chronic disease, peripheral neuropathy, affected an HIV-negative gay therapist's mobility, self-perception, relationship with his significant other, and ability to work. The author's chronic disease eventually forced him to retire from his work as a social worker in the AIDS unit of a hospital, then from his private psychotherapy practice. The article explores how the medical establishment continues to link HIV generically to the presenting medical concerns of gay men and explores the personal and collective impact of this phenomenon on gay men. *[Article copies available for a fee from The Haworth Document Delivery Service: 1-800-HAWORTH. E-mail address: <docdelivery@haworthpress.com> Website: <http://www.HaworthPress. com> © 2004 by The Haworth Press, Inc. All rights reserved.]*

KEYWORDS. Chronic illness, HIV, HIV negative, homophobia, neuropathy, psychotherapist, psychotherapy, social work

---

Charles P. Isola, MSW, can be contacted at 15 West 72nd Street #23F, New York, NY 10023-3458 (E-mail: beaujour@juno.com).

[Haworth co-indexing entry note]: "The Impact of a Non-HIV Chronic Illness on Professional Practice: Personal and Professional Considerations of a Psychotherapist." Isola, Charles P. Co-published simultaneously in *Journal of Gay & Lesbian Social Services* (Harrington Park Press, an imprint of The Haworth Press, Inc.) Vol. 17, No. 2, 2004, pp. 97-109; and: *Gay Men Living with Chronic Illnesses and Disabilities: From Crisis to Crossroads* (ed: Benjamin Lipton) Harrington Park Press, an imprint of The Haworth Press, Inc., 2004, pp. 97-109. Single or multiple copies of this article are available for a fee from The Haworth Document Delivery Service [1-800-HAWORTH, 9:00 a.m. - 5:00 p.m. (EST). E-mail address: docdelivery@ haworthpress.com].

Digital Object Identifier: 10.1300/J041v17n02_06

PROFESSIONAL HISTORY

In 1989, at 42 years of age, I left a career with a brokerage house and started social work school. After graduation, I started work as an in-patient social worker in an AIDS unit of a Manhattan hospital. When I applied for social work positions, it was the first time that I applied for a job as an out gay man. That was a terribly liberating experience for me: I was now going to be "out" not only to friends and family, but also to colleagues. The last compartment where that gay part of me was not talked about, the world of work, was going to be integrated into the rest of my life.

I felt very good about myself. I made a decision to leave, on my own terms, a career where I had earned the esteem of colleagues; I was in the fourteenth year of a solid relationship; and I had tested HIV negative from the first time I took the ELISA test. I felt that now was my time to give back to the gay community. While I had been active as a volunteer in several gay organizations from the early 1970s, in response to the AIDS crisis, I wanted to work professionally in the area of HIV. I wanted to put to use my physical energy and psychological strength to help other gay men who could directly benefit from my actions. The stamina I had had throughout my working career seemed as strong as it always had, and the psychological liberation of being "out" at work no doubt added to the physical energy and wholeness I felt about myself.

By January 1995, my work schedule consisted of 35 hours a week in the hospital, and 13 hours in private practice as a psychotherapist. I was feeling very good about myself and my work. My days were long and very active: Mornings began at 6 a.m. with gym workouts or runs, and my days ended at 9 p.m. at the end of my last session. I had energy to spare, and felt fed by both work environments.

Since my late teen years, I had continued to maintain a disciplined physical regimen of running and weightlifting, and was very cognizant of the way I looked: I did not want to reexperience the fat body I lived in until my mid-teens. I had developed a muscular "manly" body in my late teens to help cover any anxieties about appearing weak and therefore gay, and worked hard at maintaining it. (The idea that a gym body could "hide" the fact that one's body was gay worked much better in the late '60s and early '70s, when gym bodies were not as de rigeur as they are now.) When a running injury was diagnosed in late 1994, I presumed that it just "came with the territory" of having jogged for almost 25 years. It was treated with a cortisone shot. As that wore off, and the pain continued, orthotics were ordered. But they didn't help either, and I found that not only running but also walking was becoming painful. The problem became more severe, however, as I began to have difficulty stepping off curbs. Then, I found myself not able to walk a straight line. I began to "weave" as I walked down a street. In addition to the outward problems of ambulating, both feet began causing me a great deal of chronic pain, making even a sheet laying over them at night a very painful experience. As a result of these symptoms, not only walking but working was becoming very difficult.

PROCESS OF DIAGNOSIS

In June 1995, a nerve conduction study (EMG) showed peripheral nerve damage in both feet, and an MRI showed that I also had spinal stenosis–a condition where the spinal column grew together, reducing the space in the spinal canal. My doctor thought that the nerve damage was caused when the spinal column pressed in against the nerves in the canal causing the myelin around the nerves to be stripped away. This resulted in peripheral polyneuropathy which produced the chronic burning, tingling, and throbbing in both of my feet. He believed that a laminectomy, surgery to remove the extra bone, would reopen the spinal canal, and give the nerves the space they needed, allowing me to walk comfortably and also eliminate my now chronic pain. The surgery was successful, but the peripheral neuropathy pain did not decrease with either intramuscular B-12 injections or gammaglobulin IV infusions (treatments which sometimes work to reduce the pain of peripheral neuropathy).

And so the search was on for the cause of the neuropathy. Since I did not have any of the common causes of neuropathy–diabetes, chemotherapy, HIV, or HIV drugs–the cause was given as "ideopathic," or "no known cause." As I moved from doctor to doctor–GI doctors, a rheumatoid arthritis specialist, neurologists, infectious disease specialists, and internists–each one seemed to assume that the cause was HIV. There was often a quizzical look when I told them I was HIV negative. It seemed to me that there was an unspoken assumption, based on their repeatedly ordering every type of HIV test, that since I was gay, a sexually transmitted diseased had to be the cause. For me, this seemed like a case of deja vu.

In 1991, I had contracted pneumonia during a winter trip to Santa Fe. The doctor who read the X-ray wrote on his stationery that the white spot on the lung was "probably PCP since the patient is homosexual." My general practitioner showed me the note, and suggested that I have another HIV test. Although I believed at the time of that "probably PCP" diagnosis that I was HIVnegative, I did not hesitate to agree to having another ELISA HIV test.

The question still resonates: Did I really believe then that I was negative, or was there some hidden, deep conviction that since I was gay, I deserved to be/ought to be infected, and so believed I was HIV positive? And I still wonder: Was that also the unspoken thought shared by all of my health care providers as they looked for the cause of this peripheral neuropathy. And who started that unspoken dialogue between us–I or they?

As the search for a cause went on, there seemed to be a need, on the part of my doctors, to conclude that "yes, the underlying cause of this illness is sexual orientation, and therefore gay sex." So, in spite of my HIV negative status, which had, since my first HIV test in 1990, originally made me feel "safe" about what my health condition would be for the rest of my life (since I had not contracted HIV, nothing else could/would affect my health except for the common cold), there was a seeming need to put this "high-risk" category person (a gay man) into the "gay sex" cause category. And this apparent determination was shared even by those medical professionals who were themselves gay.

COURSE OF ILLNESS AND IMPACT ON PROFESSIONAL PRACTICE

I continued to work in the hospital and maintain my private practice as more blood tests were done and more neurological tests were conducted, all trying to find the cause of the neuropathy. Throughout that period, I fought to maintain my ability to work, as I began taking different pain killers to keep the neuropathic pain under control. I had to begin limiting the amount of walking I did, and had by this time stopped running or bicycling due to the intolerable pain either of those sports brought on. I had also rearranged my private practice schedule so that I had time for rest after hospital hours. The idea of reducing work hours was something I talked about in my own therapy, but at this point, between 1996 and 1998, the idea of working less due to the pain of the disease was more troubling than the actual fact of having the disease. To work less would be to admit to some kind of defeat. I was pleased with the level of competence I showed in each of my work areas, and proud of how I maintained my work schedule and my personal and professional boundaries.

I then received a call from my doctor. He informed me that my last round of blood work had come back with a T-cell count of 161. Though he did not say it, I knew that he believed that the cause had finally been confirmed: HIV. Of course, though he did not say it, I realized that if I were positive, if they found a new strain of the virus, I would now also be diagnosed with AIDS. I began telling myself very quietly that at least now I knew what the cause of my chronic pain was, and could start medications to fight the neuropathy. I left the nursing station at my job where I had taken the call, and began to wonder what drugs I would start, and how long I had to live. I unconsciously went along with the unspoken hunch of the doctors: I had a strain of HIV, and now the low T-cell count "proved" it. And all of that was due to the fact that I was gay. I had had the wrong kind of sex with the wrong kind of person.

There was a part of me that welcomed this almost certain diagnosis. While the type of disease I knew I had was diagnosed and quickly named by the results of the EMG, the cause of the illness had heretofore remained unclear, even after multiple blood workups, nerve conduction studies, tilt-table tests, GI tests, and a sural nerve biopsy (which left part of my left foot deadened). Prior to the seeming HIV diagnosis, the only treatable problem I had was a vitamin B-12 deficiency which was treatable and was reversed with intramuscular shots. As the chance of finding a treatable cause for the chronic pain disease seemed to grow more and more remote, I began to be envious of the HIV positive men I worked with at both the hospital and in my private practice. I was envious of the attention they received as a group: Drugs were being discovered and tested which helped some of them; clinical trials for people who had neuropathy as a result of HIV or HIV drugs were conducted. I tried to gain acceptance into some of those trials, but could not, since I did not have HIV. I visualized all the medical resources they had as large as a mountain. The medical resources available to me, or to people who had neuropathy, were the proverbial anthill.

The only remedies suggested were extra doses of minerals and vitamins, magnets in the soles of shoes, or TENS units (battery operated units which produced low voltage electrical charges which sometimes helped reduce pain). And of course, there was the remedy that always worked to reduce pain. This lack of remedies and lack of resources to help my problem began to wear on me. It caused me to feel envious of the men who were HIV positive: they had a disease that had a cause, and had medicines that would get them better, and hopefully keep them alive. I frequently thought of them as being "lucky." Totally irrational perhaps, but there it was.

The lack of discovery of a cause of my neuropathy left me feeling lonely and isolated even from the neuropathy community. All of the people I met at the support groups were at least 15 years older than I was, almost all were at least very overweight to obese, and all could point to a reason for their having contracted neuropathy. I also realized I was the only identified gay men or lesbian. (At the end of one meeting, an older married man came over to me and quietly told me he was gay and not out, and then asked if I had been tested for HIV. "You didn't mention that in your introduction, and that might be the cause.") The sense of being alone, being the "only one," held the same feelings I had had both as a young boy and as an adult who could not talk openly about being gay in all of my environments. I missed being part of a group. I especially missed that feeling of being complete and in control which I had when I applied for social work jobs. Then, I felt both physically and psychologically strong. Now, the chronic pain had begun to make me physically tired and psychologically unsure as to how long it would be before my health deteriorated even more.

Although my T-cell count returned to normal with the next test taken the next day, and the HIV tests continued to come back negative, the sign that my immune system was definitely compromised was something of a wake-up call. While my identification with HIV positive gay men was short-lived, it allowed me to "see" the seriousness of my disease, and convinced me to begin talking with the hospital administration about reducing my hours to two days a week at a sedentary job. Nonetheless, by the winter of 2000, the level of pain had continued to increase, even with limited movement, and I had to close my practice.

COUNTERTRANSFERENCE ISSUES WITH HIV POSITIVE GAY MEN

In my professional life as a social worker and psychotherapist, countertransference issues related to my illness shifted from when I thought I was HIV positive to when I knew for sure I was HIV negative. The first time I realized that I had not been consciously accepting the seriousness of my illness and working to integrate it into my life occurred on the same day that I received the low T-cell count from my doctor.

At the hospital, I had a new patient to meet, a gay man in his late 20s, who had been admitted the previous day. When I entered his room, he was lying in bed, propped up on a couple of pillows, his legs stretched out in front of him. He had on a hospital gown, and there was a white hospital blanket draped over his legs. His feet were sticking out from under the blanket without socks on. I walked into this room, not seeing anything unusual, just there for the business of gathering information to plan for his home care needs at discharge. I had been doing this for a long time, walking into a scene like this one, and I entered the space with no sense of how important that meeting was going to be for me.

He was a good looking young man, and, as often happened to me at these moments, I thought to myself that he was cute. Dark hair combed over his head to the side, rather long and curly at the end. He was thin but did not "look" sick. I said my usual hello, and after the preliminary introductions, sat in a chair at the foot of the bed, just opposite his feet. He lived alone and never had needed help after his prior hospital discharges. Today, however, he was concerned about going home and being alone since his neuropathy was getting so painful. It was making it almost impossible to walk, let alone stand. I was surprised at his mention of the word. (How strong denial is: After I left the room I reread his chart and the neuropathy was mentioned quite a few times.) I suddenly felt myself become very close to him. "Oh, is that why the blanket is off your feet?" I felt emotionally overwhelmed when he said it was. My mind went on autopilot and I heard myself telling him that I too knew what it was like to not be able to keep the blanket on your feet, to wake up several times during the night from burning feet hanging off the bed in search of someplace comfortable.

He looked at me rather incredulously and asked if I had neuropathy. "Yes," I answered, feeling very close and warm towards him. He looked surprised and sounded sad when he said, "But I guess it isn't as bad as mine." I immediately felt embarrassed and foolish. Here I was, a few minutes after walking unassisted into the room, sitting there with shoes on, telling him I had the same illness he had. A minute prior I had felt so connected to him, so understanding of what he was going through. Now I wanted nothing more than to be able to run away from him, his feet, his pain, his neuropathy, and any other questions he might ask. He might ask me another question about me. He might ask if I were positive, and even though that morning I began to think that I was, at that moment, dreading the next question, I really did not want to join with anyone who was HIV positive in a disease-related way. I wanted nothing to do with the possibility that we were too much alike in our diseases. And if he asked, what would I say? "Yes, maybe." "I think so?" "Well, we'll see, they're still testing?"

Luckily for me at that moment, he did not ask. But after the realization of what I had done in that meeting began to sink in, and when the results of the new HIV and T-cell count came back, I found that I began to distance myself from my HIV positive patients. During supervision sessions I realized that my own health concerns were impacting negatively on my clinical work. I became more protective and less challenging of my patients' maladaptive defenses which mirrored my own. As I protected myself from my own fears, I unwittingly protected these clients from helping them to look into their own fears and issues–whether or not they were HIV related.

COUNTERTRANSFERENCE ISSUES
WITH HIV NEGATIVE MEN

Even as I was protecting my HIV positive patients, I found myself beginning to trivialize the problems (especially health-related issues) that HIVnegative patients brought in, and as my ability to ambulate became more painful, my concerns about my body image increased. The thought of becoming the weak, fat me of my teens became frightening, and totally at odds with the "always healthy" way my life was going to be when I received that first HIVnegative diagnosis. After all, since I was a partner in a stable, long-term relationship and had dodged HIV, didn't happiness and contentment have to be in my future?

A year before I finally decided to close my practice due to an increasing fatigue, a former client called and wanted to return to therapy. He was twenty years younger than I, and overweight. He originally left therapy about 18 months before, due to financial problems, especially caused by what he had considered to be my overly expensive fee. The individual in question was someone in whom I recognized too many unwanted parts of myself which I had for years tried to split off, but had gradually and very grudgingly come to accept–or so I had thought.

At the time he called to resume therapy, I needed several naps during the day to keep my energy level up. When he walked into my office, my first thought was that he had put on a lot of weight. Whether he had or not was not the issue, but as I looked at him, I could feel a vacuum develop in the room; his neediness felt like it had grown, no doubt in direct proportion to how huge I believed he had become. Before he started talking, whatever energy and interest I had in working with him was pulled out of me. His battles with religion, with boyfriends, with family, the constant searching for acceptance in places that would never grant it, his unending anger at any authority figure were back. I listened. I felt tired. At the end of the session, he said it felt good to be back. It was as if he had said nothing. I heard my voice saying, in a matter-of-fact tone, that my fee had increased since the last time I saw him, and that the new fee schedule would start next week. I apologized for having failed to tell him about the increase on the phone. He looked at me rather blankly, no doubt with the same expression that was on my face, stood up, paid me for the session, and walked out the door.

As he closed the door, it struck me that I had enacted something, but at the moment I couldn't quite place what I had done. I did, however, instinctively realize that he would not be back. While I felt concern for this man, I also felt relief for me, knowing that he would not return and I would not be confronted with the image of what I was most afraid of becoming—helpless, dependent, needy, unattractive. It was soon after that incident that I realized I needed to rethink my own abilities as a therapist, and to begin paying more attention to the reality of my disease, especially as it was affecting my ability to manage feelings and continue to do effective psychotherapy.

DISCLOSURE CONCERNS

At the end of the summer, 1999, after long discussions in therapy, with colleagues, and with my partner, I reached the decision to close my private practice. I was becoming more worn down by the painkillers and the pain, and did not have the real energy I needed to do my work. I decided to stop work in February of 2000, but wanted to present my decision early enough to give each patient ample time to explore feelings about termination, without having it coincide too closely with the holidays which usually produced their own conflicted sets of emotions. So, I decided that I would begin each session that first week of November with the announcement that I was closing my practice at the end of February due to personal issues.

I decided that if there were any questions specifically asking why I was leaving my practice, I would explain the medical problem that required this decision. Given that the majority of my gay patients had heard of neuropathy, I was also ready to be asked and to disclose my HIV status should they ask that question. I felt very comfortable with that strategy for my gay patients. However, I did not feel comfortable discussing my health issues with any of the four straight patients I was working with (one woman, three men) at the time. Three already knew I was gay. The other man had never asked, though I was certain that he knew. I somehow imagined that this very bright and articulate man in his thirties, whose parents were doctors, knew what was wrong with me, since he had never seen me with shoes on (I had worked in socks since 1995 in order to keep the level of pain to a minimum).

In the weeks leading up to disclosing that I would be closing my practice, I was becoming more and more anxious about the questions these four people would ask, particularly this man. The anxiety was palpable. I fantasized that even though I knew that what I would be saying was the truth–that I had idiopathic neuropathy–somehow he would be able to tell I was lying by the guilty look on my face. I realized that someplace deep within me, I still held the belief that I was really not all right, neither physically or morally, due to the indelible stigma of being gay.

The session with this patient went as I thought it would; he asked if I knew what the cause was. I told him it was an ideopathic neuropathy. I was surprised at his reaction: an uncle had gotten the disease after becoming diabetic. He expressed his hope that it wouldn't become too painful. He even mentioned that his uncle had gotten some relief from gammaglobulin, and hoped it would work for me. He then continued to talk about his issues.

I think back to this case, and see it as my own internalized homophobia still there, still alive as I presented my gay self to this heterosexual man. He was a "real" man. I was a sickly fake. The feelings of sickness and guilt I had about myself as a young boy, which I tried to cover with the manly, muscular body, were back, and still as strong as they were some forty years before. It is a bit frightening to me, as I write this, seven years after that session took place, how this question of "realness" and masculinity affected me as a 7-year-old, and then again when the neuropathy was diagnosed, and throughout my life as a gay therapist and gay man. That young boy I once was had a very hard time believing that he was a real boy, and that early imprinted belief continued to work its twisted logic on me, even as I considered how this patient would react to my disclosure of an illness.

RELATIONSHIP ISSUES

After the peripheral neuropathy diagnosis, as I learned more about the illness, I became increasingly fearful that my sensory neuropathy would turn into a motor disease which might impinge on my ability to walk. As I talked with my partner of now 25 years about the possibilities of this happening, I wondered out loud, not really intending it to be a direct question to him: "What if I can't walk someday?" And he replied, "I'll carry you." My immediate reaction was relief, happiness, sadness, then fear. The "relief" and "happiness" were to know that he would stay with me and carry me. The fear was twofold; first, that I might lose my ability to walk; and second, that I might actually become physically dependent on my partner. How wonderful it was for me that he would be there; how horrible that I might need him to be.

At that moment, my partner had become more important to me; not only would I depend on him for love and emotional support, but now there was the distinct possibility that I would become physically dependent on him as well. I thought that I had accepted this prospect of a new kind of dependence as yet another sign of the love and trust we had for each other. I felt very proud of myself, being able to accept the offer he made, the sympathy he showed for me. But the deeper feelings of fear which I didn't realize were there, surfaced one evening as I was leading a group for gay men in my practice.

Several months before I made the final decision to close my practice, due to my increasing fatigue and reliance on painkillers, I walked into the room to begin the session. As I sat down, one of the group members whom I liked very much asked, "So, who's downstairs?" Since its beginning, when any member of the group asked about the apartment, or wondered about whom it was I lived with, I would also ask that member to talk about what their fantasy was about us. I remember feeling angry at something–at the moment I didn't know what–and answered quickly, even as I settled into the chair, "His name is Bill." The group was silent for a moment, and someone made the comment, "So at least we know it's a 'he.'" There was laughter at the comment; I said, "Yes, it's a 'he.'" There was silence again. I wondered out loud if there were any other questions about me (I fantasized that they knew I was ill). One group member said he would rather talk about himself, and the group moved on.

I brought my comment into supervision and my own therapy. I found myself saying that I had "flung" the answer into the middle of the group, but I couldn't figure out why I would use that verb or why I felt so smug as I said it. As I teased out the emotions that had led me to make the statement, I discovered that the smugness came from the fact that I was the only person in the room who was in a relationship, and I felt superior to the members about that. Group members had often addressed my being coupled, sometimes with anger, sometimes with envy, but I had never been in touch with this newfound smugness. I realized that the "flinging" was about a fear that they, or anyone, might come between me and my partner. I wanted my relationship off limits to everyone; there should be no wondering about it; no questioning of it. There was to be no interference from anyone in the relationship with the person who might have to carry me; it was difficult enough that I was even allowing myself to think about being carried. I wanted to shut them and everyone else out. I must have done a pretty good job of it, since there were no more comments about him or the apartment during the next seven months that the group met.

CONCLUSION

Now 56 years old and several years after facing the challenges outlined in this chapter, I feel a strange mixture of relief and incredulity. I feel the relief that comes from accepting the fact that there will likely not be a cure for my disease for many years. I've tried herbs, diet change, acupuncture, reflexology, massage, yoga, and meditation, and have finally factored my disease into being an ongoing part of my life. Barring an unexpected medical breakthrough, I believe that I will live with chronic pain for the rest of my life. I am hopeful that the disease will remain sensory, and not become an autonomic or motor neuropathy that could attack internal organs or destroy my muscles and sense of balance. Approaching the eighth year since my initial diagnosis, if I have not made a real "peace" with my disease, I have at least ceded it a place within my body.

My incredulity arises from several different sources. The first is at my unconscious belief that since I had escaped HIV infection, I would also be immune from the many other illnesses that routinely affect all people as they age. My disavowal was in no way do to lack of exposure to illness or the effects of aging. I had volunteered with Senior Action in Gay Environment since my late 20s, and my first long-term relationship had been with a man 40 years older than I. Rather, I think my belief that avoiding HIV equaled a long and healthy life is part of the deep and traumatic effect that HIV and AIDS continues to have on the gay community. If my disavowal is, in fact, indicative of other HIV negative gay men, then social service professionals working with men of my generation not only will find themselves dealing with patients facing universal aging issues, but also with gay-specific feelings of confusion and anger: "I've been 'good' for so long, and didn't contract the virus. How can this other illness be happening to me now?"

My incredulity also relates to my willingness to go along with medical professionals in so desperately trying to find that the cause of my disease was HIV related. This speaks, I believe, to a deeply ingrained, internalized homophobia in our medical system that pervades gay and straight providers alike. I also believe that my own internal self-loathing still asserted that I was not quite as morally good as a "normal" heterosexual person. My being homosexual required punishment somehow: a doctor would surmise that a spot on a lung X-ray must be PCP, or repeatedly order T-cell counts because I just had to be HIV positive. I succumbed to the belief that homosexuality equaled degeneracy equaled HIV.

After so much psychological work on myself, how is it possible that the self-loathing was still there? How ingrained is it still in other (maybe all) gay men? I think too many of us have assumed that if we really strived vigilantly for self-awareness, we could undo most, if not all, of the centuries of oppression that preceded the mere three and a half decades since Stonewall. Upon reflection, I wonder now if I had been attuned enough to the role that internalized homophobia played in my gay patients' therapy: Was I able to help them approach theirs, if I had trouble approaching my own?

Finally, there is the incredulity about the very "realness" of my pain. Prior to the official diagnosis of neuropathy, before the medical establishment put a word to it, I wondered constantly if, in fact, my pain was real. Was there just a "touch" of hypochondria going on? Prior to the onset of my illness, I know that there were times when I would doubt others complaints of pain if there was no medically proven cause of it. What does that say about my need (and perhaps society's in general) to have my subjectivity validated by an "expert"? How can we, as service providers, utilize diagnostic categories as useful supports in treatment planning versus tools of validation or dismissal?

Writing this article has brought back in painfully vivid detail the effects of my disease on both my life course and my sense of self. It has also reinforced the importance of seeing myself as a person with agency who has an affect on how his disease is defined. I am hopeful that my story will help practicing clinicians in their work with gay men, both HIV negative and HIV positive, who are forced to deal with the difficult challenges related to chronic illnesses and disabilities.

Index

Adolescents, gay, coping strategies of, 11-12
ADRESSING model (Hays), 36
Advocacy, social service providers and, 18-19
Aging, 82-83
  coping with chronic illness and, 17-18
  impact of AIDS, 84-85
  loss and, 83-84
  oppression of, within gay communities, 86-87
  study of gay gerontology and, 83-84
AIDS. *See also* HIV
  impact of, aging and, 84-85
  stigma and, 8
Americans with Disabilities Act (ADA), 30-31
Apathy, HIV positive gay men and, 71-72

Best practices, in mental health, 33-36
Body, sociocultural theories of, 48-53
  disability theory, 51-53
  feminist theories, 48-49
  poststructuralist theories, 49-51
  queer theory, 51
Body image disturbance. *See also* Gay beauty
  gay men and, 45-47,57-60
  overview of, 44-45

Change, advocating, 18-19

Chronic illnesses. *See also* Illnesses; Non-HIV chronic illnesses (NHIVCIs)
  adjusting to diagnosis of, 3-4
  defining, 3
  diagnosis of, 3
  effect of, on people, 3
  incidence and prevalence of, among gay men, 2-3
  psychotherapy interventions for gay men with, 34
  social construction of, 6-8
Cognitive deterioration, HIV positive gay men and, 68
Coming out process, 9
Coping strategies
  gay adolescents and, 11-12
  for gay men living with NHIVCIs, 12-13
  social support as, 12-13
Countertransference issues, with HIV positive gay men, 102-104
Cult of masculinity, 55-56
Cultural imperialism, 87-88

Death, therapists and issues of, 77
Disabilities. *See also* Gay men living with NHIVCIs
  vs. handicaps, 32-33
  identity development process for persons with, 29
  impact of, on sexual functioning, 34-35
  social construction approaches to, 30
  universal essentialist approach to, 32
Disability identity, development of, 29

Disability Identity Attitude Scale
(DIAS), 29-30
Disability theory, 51-53
Discrimination
minority gay men with disabilities
and, 28
stigma of, 17
Diseases, describing, 3
Diversity, ethnocultural, gay men
living with NHIVCIs and,
16-17
Double consciousness, 88

Effeminancy, history of, 53-54
Empowerment, promoting, 15
Ethnocultural diversity, gay men living
with NHIVCIs and, 16-17

Feminist theories, of the body, 48-49
Foucault, M., 49-50
Friend, R. A., 82-83

Gay adolescents, coping strategies and,
11-12
Gay beauty. *See also* Body image
disturbance
history of, 53-54
subculture of, 54-56
Gay gerontology, study of, 83-84
Gay identity
formation spectrum of, 82-83, 91
positive, and social support, 12
social constructions of, 6-8,30
Gay men. *See also* HIV negative gay
men; HIV positive gay men
ageist oppression by, 86-87
body image disturbance among,
45-47
discrimination and, 28
gender oppression among, 57-60
heterosexual medical providers
and, 5

incidence and prevalence of chronic
illnesses among, 2-3
perception of social supports and,
13
specter of HIV for, and diagnosis of
chronic illness, 4
Gay men living with disabilities. *See*
Gay men living with
NHIVCIs
Gay men living with NHIVCIs. *See
also* Non-HIV chronic
illnesses (NHIVCIs)
coping strategies for, 12-13
disclosing information to medical
providers and, 35-36
guidelines for supporting, 13-19
advocating change, 18-19
aging and, 17-18
promoting empowerment, 15
promoting group work, 15-16
recognizing legacy of pathology,
13-14
responding to ethnocultural
diversity, 16-17
guilt and, 35
intervention strategies and
techniques for, 36-37
minority, discrimination and, 28
physical overvaluation/idealization
and, 35
psychotherapy interventions for, 34
sexual functioning and, 34-35
stigma and, 8-11
Gender oppression, among gay men,
57-60
Group identity, positive
positive self-perceptions and, 12
Guilt, gay men living with NHIVCIs
and, 35

Handicaps, *vs.* disabilities, 32-33
Health care workers, homophobia and
heterosexism among, 18

Heterosexism, among health care
    workers, 18
HIV, specter of, for gay men, 4-5. *See
    also* AIDS
HIV drug-related side effects, 66-67
HIV negative gay men,
    countertransference issues
    with, 104-105. *See also* Gay
    men
HIV positive gay men. *See also* Gay men
    change in social status and, 70-71
    countertransference issues with,
        102-104
    factors complicating psychotherapy
        with, 72-77
    fear of cognitive deterioration and, 68
    HIV drug-related side effects and,
        66-67
    overview of changes in issues for,
        64-66
    stigmatization and, 68-70
Homophobia, among health care
    workers, 18
Homosexuality, shifts in social
    constructions of, 7-8

Identity. *See* Gay identity
Illnesses. *See also* Chronic illnesses
    describing, 3
    impact of, on sexual functioning,
        34-35
    social construction of, 7

Labeling, 9-10
"Learning to hide" coping strategy,
    11-12
Lipodystrophy, 68-69
Loss, aging and, 84-85, 85

Marginalization, 86

Masculinity, cult of, 55-56
Medical providers
    disclosing information to, gay men
        and, 35-36
    gay men and, 5
    homophobia and heterosexism
        among, 18
Mental health, best practices in, 33-36
Mental health providers
    clients with disabilities and, 33-34
    intervention strategies and
        techniques for, 36-37
Minorities
    defined, 27
    healthy identity development for,
        29-31
    sociological, 27-29
Minority gay men with disabilities,
    discrimination and, 28
Minority status, minority stress and,
    11-12
Minority stress, 9
    minority status and, 11-12

NHIVCIs. *See* Non-HIV chronic
    illnesses (NHIVCIs)
Non-HIV chronic illnesses (NHIVCIs),
    2. *See also* Chronic illnesses;
    Gay men living with
    NHIVCIs
    biopsychosocial definition of, 3-6
    example of impact of, on
        psychotherapist's
        professional practice,
        98-102,108-109
    no-man's land for gay men living
        with, 6
    organizational support for gay men
        living with, 5-6
    stigma and gay men living with, 8-11
Nursing students, homophobia and
    heterosexism among, 18

Pathology, recognizing legacy of, 13-14
Physicians, male, homophobia and
    heterosexism among, 18
Poststructuralist theories, of the body,
    49-51
Providers. *See* Medical providers;
    Mental health providers;
    Social service providers
Psychotherapists
    countertransference issues for,
        102-105
    disclosure concerns for, 105-106
    example of impact of NHIVCI on
        professional practice of,
        98-102
    relationship issues for, 106-108
Psychotherapists, HIV positive gay
    men and, 77-78
Psychotherapy
    challenges of, for therapists, 77-78
    factors complicating, with HIV
        positive gay men, 72-77

Queer theory, of the body, 51

Self-perceptions, positive group
    identity and, 12
Senior Action in a Gay Environment
    (SAGE), 82-83,93-94,108
    case example of intervention by,
        90-93
    intervention strategies of, 88-90
Sexual functioning, impact of
    illness/disability on, 34-35
Sexual identity formation, model of,
    82-83, 91
Social constructions
    of disabilities, 30
    of gay identity, 30

people with chronic illnesses and,
    31
Social model of disability, 52
Social service providers, advocacy for
    change and, 18-19
Social status, HIV positive gay men
    and, 70-71
Social supports
    as coping strategy, 12-13
    perception of, by gay men, 13
Sociological minorities, 27-29
Stigma
    AIDS and, 8
    concept of, 9
    of discrimination, 17
    gay men living with NHIVCIs and,
        8-11
    impact of, and gay men living with
        NHIVCIs, 10-11
    people with illnesses and, 9-10
    vigilance and, 11-12
Stigmatization, 9-10
    HIV positive gay men and, 68-70
Stress. *See* Minority stress
Support groups, gay men living with
    NHIVICs and, 16
Survivor guilt, 4

Therapists. *See* Psychotherapists

Universal essentialist approach, to
    disabilities, 32

Vigilance, stigma and, 11-12

Wilde, Oscar, 54

*For Product Safety Concerns and Information please contact
our EU representative GPSR@taylorandfrancis.com Taylor & Francis
Verlag GmbH, Kaufingerstraße 24, 80331 München, Germany*

T - #0128 - 160425 - C0 - 212/152/8 - PB - 9781560233367 - Gloss Lamination